Connective Tissue Disease - Current State of the Art

Edited by Akira Takeda

Published in London, United Kingdom

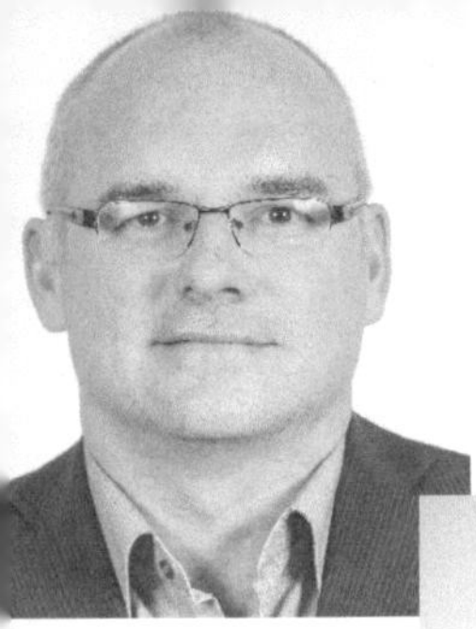
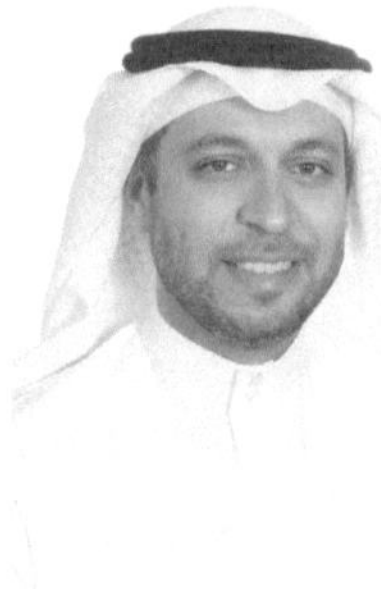
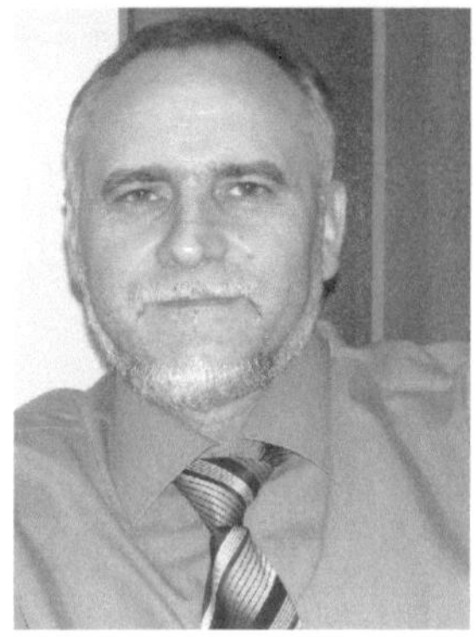
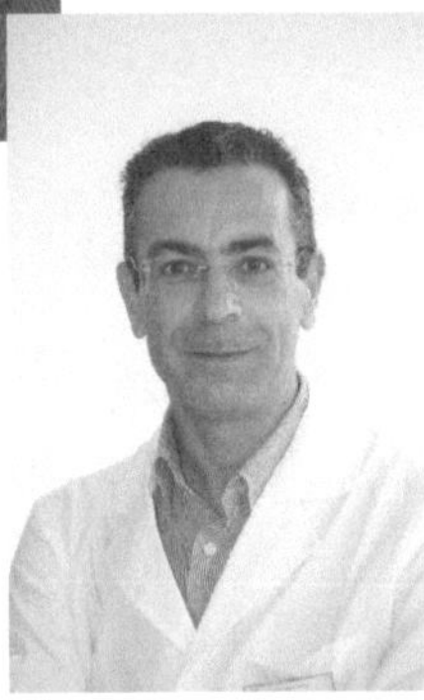
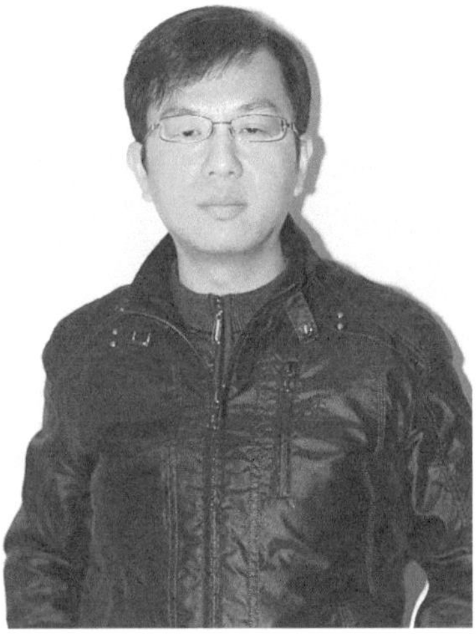
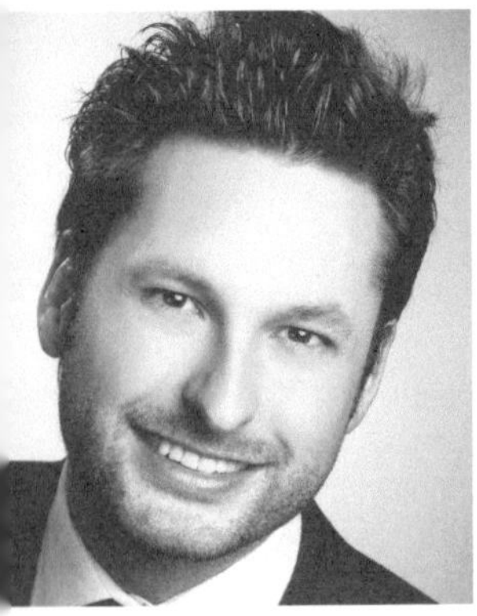
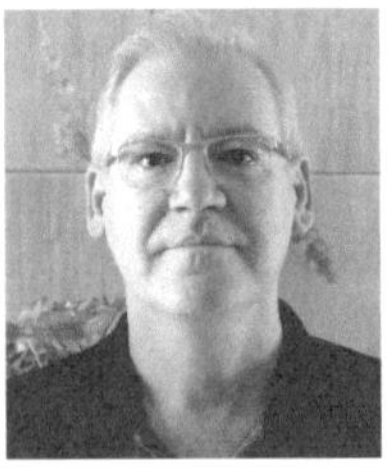

IntechOpen

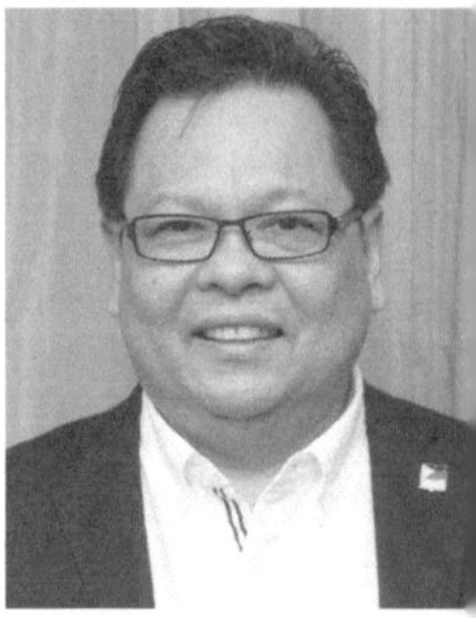
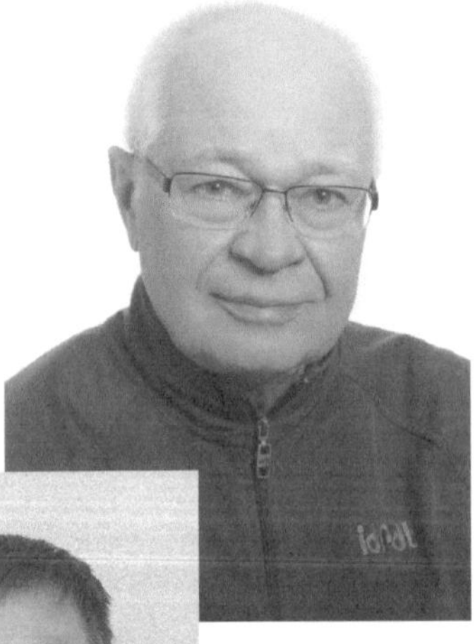
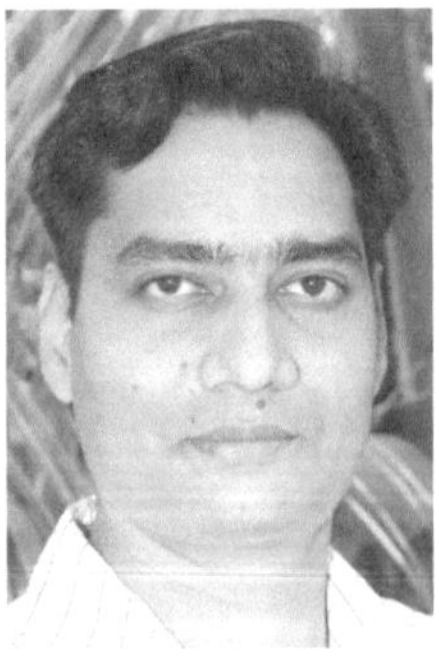
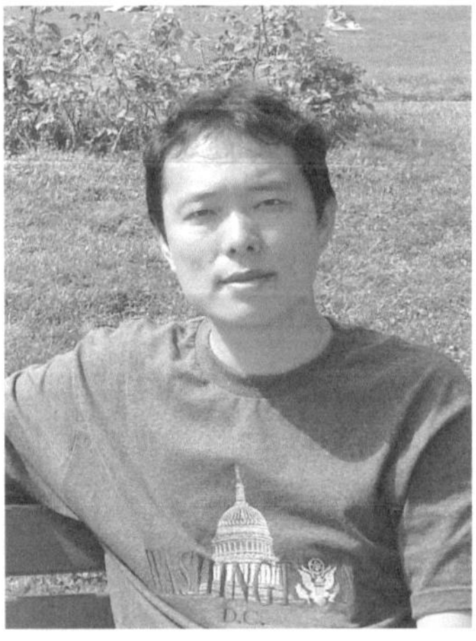
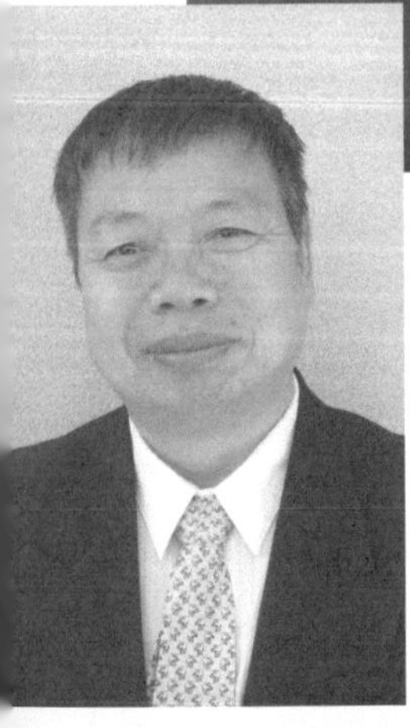
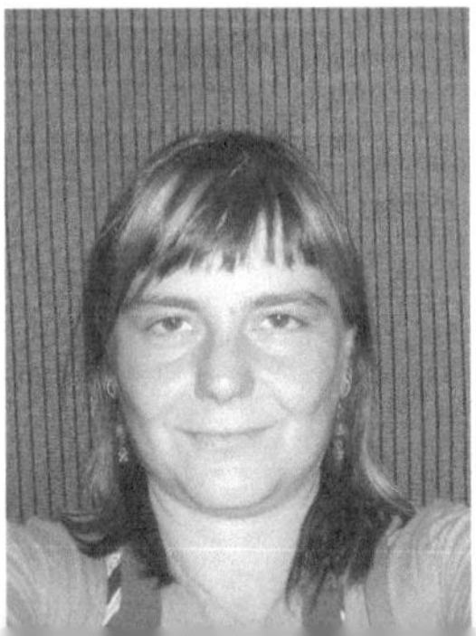

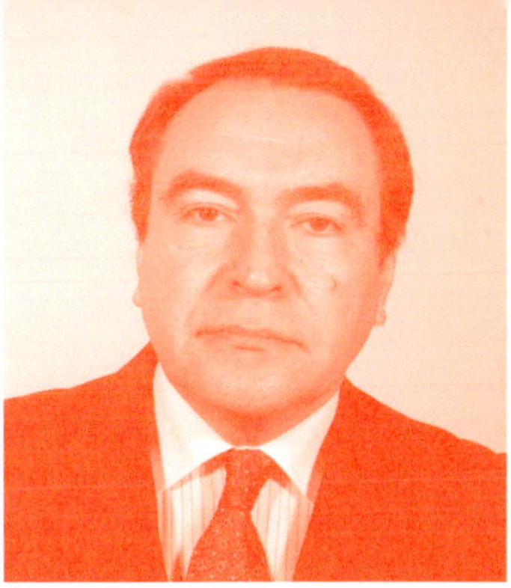
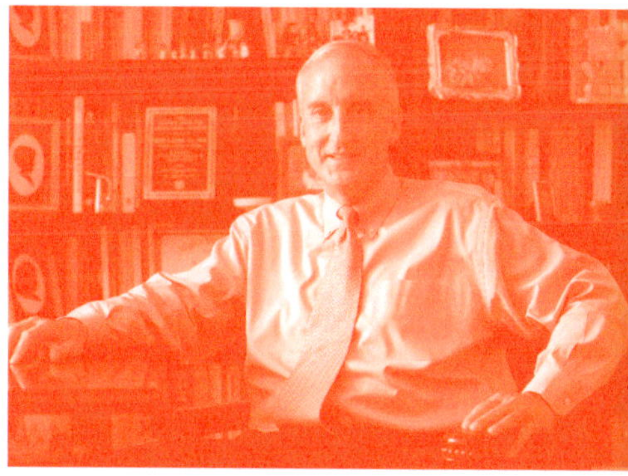
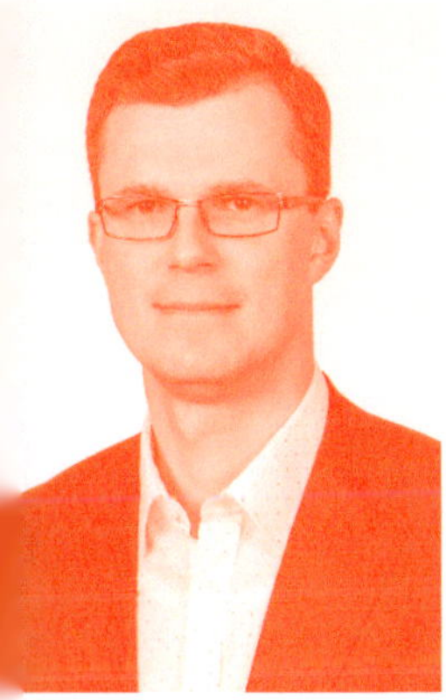
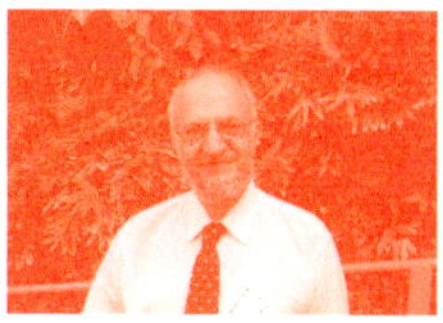
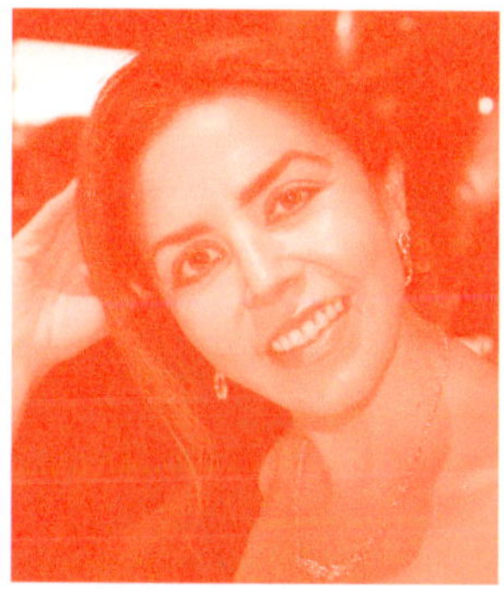

Supporting open minds since 2005

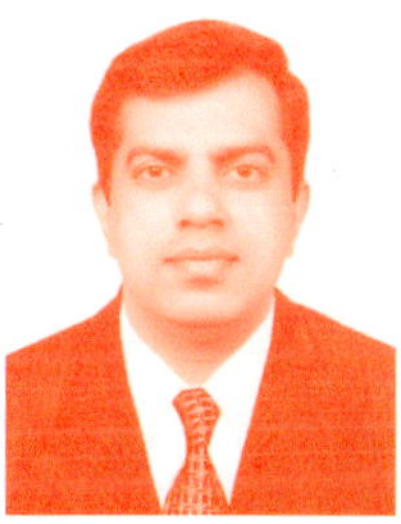
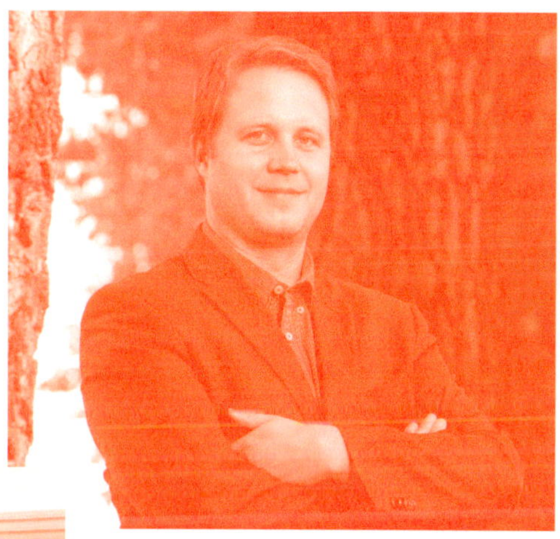
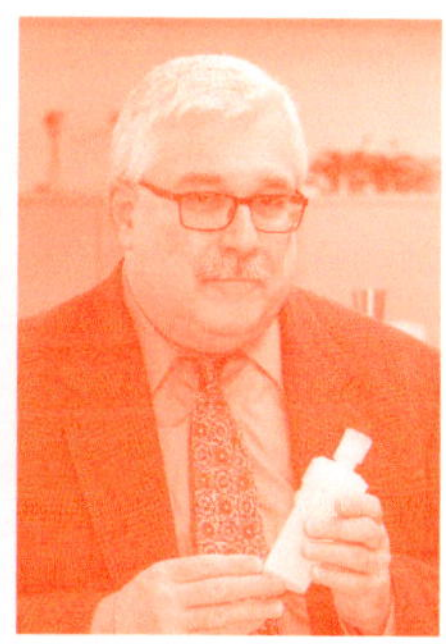
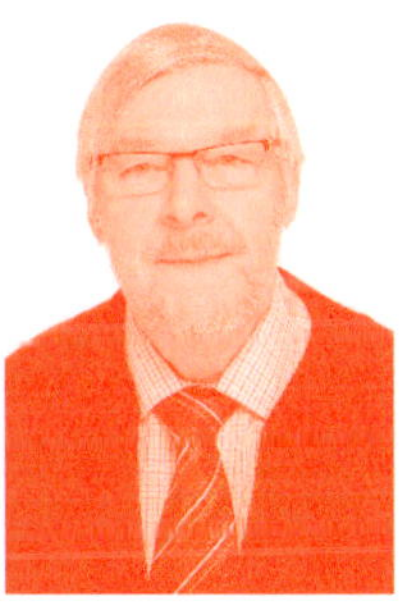
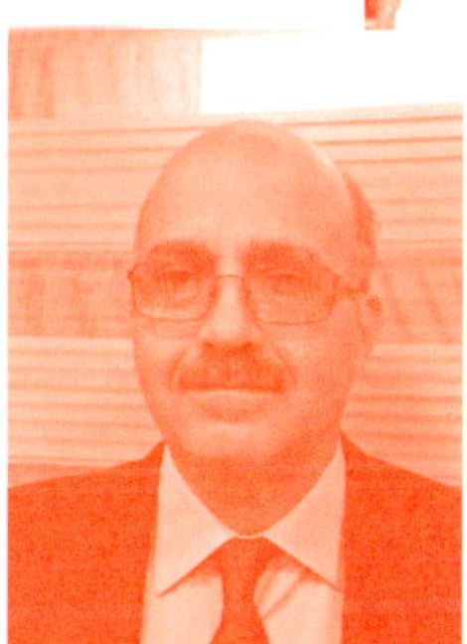
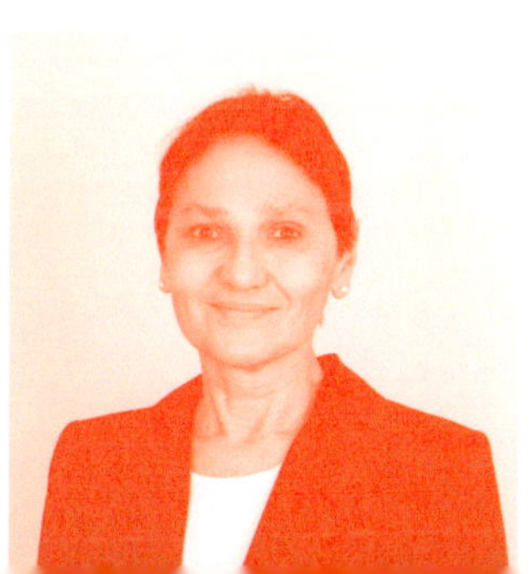
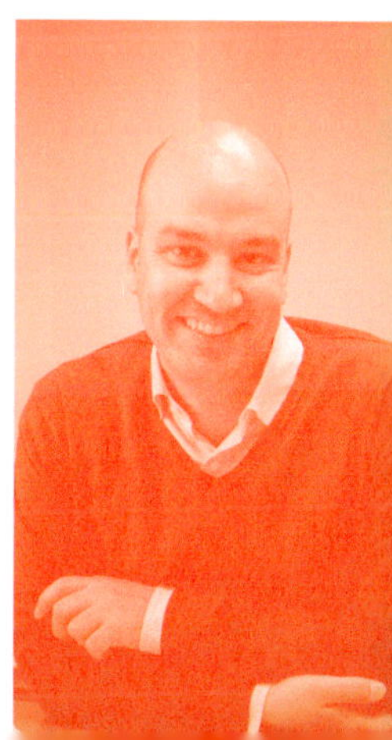

Connective Tissue Disease - Current State of the Art
http://dx.doi.org/10.5772/intechopen.76664
Edited by Akira Takeda

Contributors
Balaji Zacharia, Antony Roy, Ricardo Munir Nahas, Vivianne Hosti Dos Santos, Silvio Lopes Alabarse, Matthew Parker, Neil McGill, Xin Ran, Yuping Ran, Peng Wang, Jinghong Huang, Sushmita Pradhan, Akira Takeda, Hideharu Sugimoto, Yang Heli

First published in London, United Kingdom, 2020 by IntechOpen
IntechOpen is the global imprint of INTECHOPEN LIMITED, registered in England and Wales, registration number: 11086078, 7th floor, 10 Lower Thames Street, London, EC3R 6AF, United Kingdom
Printed in Croatia

British Library Cataloguing-in-Publication Data
A catalogue record for this book is available from the British Library

Additional hard and PDF copies can be obtained from orders@intechopen.com

Connective Tissue Disease - Current State of the Art
Edited by Akira Takeda
p. cm.
Print ISBN 978-1-78985-698-9
Online ISBN 978-1-78985-841-9
eBook (PDF) ISBN 978-1-78985-842-6

Meet the editor

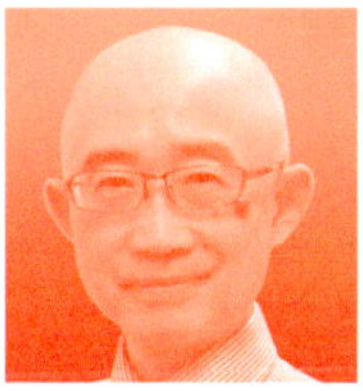

Akira Takeda, MD, PhD, is the founder and director of the Division of Clinical Immunology & Rheumatology at International University of Health and Welfare Hospital, Japan. He graduated from Akita University School of Medicine, Japan, after which he joined Jichi Medical School, where he was actively involved in clinical rheumatology practice as well as basic research in the field of Immunology. After completing his thesis studies, he worked as an assistant professor at the University of Massachusetts Medical School while pursuing extensive studies of cellular and humoral immunity against pathogens to elucidate the precise host defense mechanisms. Upon his return to Japan, Dr. Takeda joined Dokkyo University School of Medicine and the current institute where he has been exploring the immuno-pathogenesis of connective tissue disease (CTD)-associated organ injury, leading to numerous publications including novel research into how T cells trigger and promote interstitial pneumonia in CTDs.

Contents

Preface

Connective tissue diseases (CTDs) constitute a heterogenous group of systemic autoimmune disorders and related conditions, characterized by rheumatic manifestations, production of myriad autoantibodies, and varied immune-mediated organ injury. Included in this category are rheumatoid arthritis (RA), systemic lupus erythematosus (SLE), scleroderma (systemic sclerosis; SSc), polymyositis/dermatomyositis (PM/DM), systemic vasculitides, and Sjögren's syndrome (SS), among others. During the past few decades, a great paradigm shift has occurred in the realm of therapeutics due to advances in our understanding of disease etiopathology. Robust emerging evidence on the precise role of the innate and adaptive immune systems and their contributions to initiation and development of CTDs has facilitated our understanding of disease, generating great interest in immunotherapy including numerous biologics. To achieve the best outcomes for patients, timely and accurate evaluation has become fundamental and, as such, advanced diagnostic and assessment modalities have also been developed, and have had a revolutionary impact in precise characterization of the disease conditions in CTDs.

Connective Tissue Disease: Current State of the Art consists of five chapters that combine systematic reviews, investigations and original clinical studies; comprehensive rheumatologic perspectives on RA, lupus and the other arthritides such as spondyloarthritis; new concepts of diagnostic modalities; and clinical implications of physical therapy. In Chapter 1, which serves as an introductory chapter and which has original material, we start with a comprehensive overview of the recent and revolutionary paradigm shift in RA, the most common of the CTDs, emphasizing the urgent need for diagnostic precision. This leads us to the introduction of our proposed "diagnostic criteria for early RA with MRI findings." Chapter 2 discusses lupus, the most typical of the systemic autoimmune disease in its ability to cause widespread inflammation and tissue damage in affected organs including skin, joints, brain, lungs, kidneys, and blood vessels. The authors provide intriguing dermatologic perspectives based on their studies with dermoscopy and histopathology. Chapter 3 elegantly demonstrates recent advances in nail fold capillaroscopy, a modality that is extremely important today in the evaluation of patients with Raynaud's phenomenon and systemic sclerosis (SSc) spectrum diseases. Considering that vasculature changes by functional and structural alterations of the microcirculation play a central role in the pathogenesis of CTDs, this methodology gives new impetus for improvement of precision evaluation of disease in daily practice. Chapter 4 covers the disease concept of spondyloarthritis (SpA) in which several subtypes can be distinguished, including ankylosing spondylitis (AS), psoriatic arthritis (PsA), SpA related to inflammatory bowel disease (IBD-SpA), reactive arthritis (ReA), and undifferentiated SpA (uSpA). Chapter 5 appraises the increasing importance of physical activity and exercise training in the clinical course of CTDs, explaining the benefits of exercise on physical limitations and fatigue in these diseases, with both short- and long-term effectiveness.

Written by expert clinical and research scientists who are directly involved in patient care and CTD research, this book covers a broad spectrum of interests and provide a deep understanding of this category of diseases for rheumatologists, physician scientists, researchers, and students. I would like to extend my heartfelt appreciation to all the authors for their time and effort in providing their best, and Ms. Sara Debeuc at IntechOpen for her diligent editorial assistance. Additionally, I am grateful to Hideharu Sugimoto, MD, my old colleague, a radiology expert at Jichi Medical University School of Medicine, for fruitful long-term collaborations and discussions. Finally, I would like to convey special thanks to Professor Gautam A. Deshpande, MD, at the Department of General Medicine, Juntendo University, for his sapient advice and vital support throughout the process of compilation. His encouragement made it possible to achieve the goal.

Akira Takeda, MD, PhD
Division of Clinical Immunology and Rheumatology,
International University of Health and Welfare Hospital,
Nasu-Shiobara, Tochigi, Japan

Chapter 1

Growing Need for Diagnostic Precision in Rheumatoid Arthritis: Proposal of MR Imaging Criteria for Early Diagnosis

Akira Takeda and Hideharu Sugimoto

Abstract

The recent and revolutionary paradigm shift involving novel therapeutics for the treatment of rheumatoid arthritis (RA) has called for changes in the early diagnosis of RA. Physicians now need to diagnose RA earlier, and with greater accuracy, in order to initiate effective definitive treatment as early as possible. However, due to the complexity and diverseness of RA, we still do not have comprehensive diagnostic criteria for RA readily available. To find a solution to this challenge, we aimed to develop practically useful criteria which integrate gadolinium (Gd) contrast-enhanced magnetic resonance imaging (MRI) findings with clinical manifestations of the disease. These diagnostic criteria we propose, the "diagnostic criteria for early RA with MRI findings," are composed of two domains. The first domain consists of clinical findings suggestive of RA, which include both entry criteria—i.e., polyarthralgia of hands (joint pain of three or more joint areas confirmed by a physician), and exclusion criteria—i.e., exclusion of other rheumatic conditions including systemic lupus erythematosus (SLE), dermatomyositis and polymyositis (PM/DM), mixed connective tissue disease (MCTD), primary Sjögren's syndrome (SS), and Behçet's disease (BD). The second domain constitutes MRI criteria, which represent Gd-enhanced MRI findings indicating bilateral synovial enhancement seen in any joints of the proximal interphalangeal (PIP), metacarpophalangeal (MCP), or wrist joints. RA is defined by fulfilling all conditions of both domains. Our prospective study demonstrated that these criteria for the diagnosis of early RA, incorporating MRI findings with physical manifestations, can successfully distinguish patients with RA from those with other mimicking conditions, showing a sensitivity of 96%, specificity of 86%, and accuracy of 92%. When a case does not meet the criteria, RA can be ruled out with a high negative predictive value of 95%. We believe our "diagnostic criteria for early RA with MRI findings" can greatly help to solve unmet diagnostic needs in the early treatment of RA.

Keywords: rheumatoid arthritis (RA), early RA, magnetic resonance imaging (MRI), gadolinium (Gd) contrast-enhanced MRI, diagnostic criteria

1. Introduction

Rheumatoid arthritis (RA), an autoimmune systemic inflammatory disease marked by progressive joint destruction, disability, and mortality, is the most common connective tissue disease (CTD), occurring in 1–2% of the population, and more frequently in women. The disease is primarily characterized by synovial inflammation which leads to an erosive/destructive polyarthropathy, predominantly affecting the peripheral joints, but also with extra-articular manifestations including subcutaneous nodules, skin ulceration, scleritis/episcleritis, pericarditis, splenomegaly, and a variety of pleuro-pulmonary disorders which may develop during its clinical course.

1.1 Etiology

Although the etiology of RA has not yet been fully elucidated, it is recognized as a multifactorial disease associated with genetic susceptibility, environmental triggering, hormonal predisposition, and possibly infections. Genetic risk factors include human leukocyte antigen (HLA)-DR4, in particular, HLA–DRB1 alleles encoding a common amino acid sequence (the "shared epitope") in the third hypervariable region of the DRB1 molecule [1]. The HLA-DRB1*04 alleles (HLA-DRB1*0401, *0404, *0408, and *0405) show the strongest association with RA, especially with anti-citrullinated protein antibody (ACPA)-positive RA [2]. These alleles have in common a highly conserved sequence between amino acids 67 and 74 along the α-helix derived from the DRβ chain, which forms one side of the antigen-binding site of the DR molecule [3]. Studies have shown that the shared epitope alleles may preferably present citrullinated peptides [4]. In addition to the HLA locus, recent genome-wide association studies (GWAS) have revealed many high-risk RA susceptibility genes, such as *CD244*, *PADI4*, *SLC22A2*, *PTPN22*, *CTLA4*, and *STAT4* [5]. However, except for some loci, the function of most of these RA risk loci remains unclear.

Among multiple environmental and behavioral risk factors that have been studied, cigarette smoking is identified as the strongest trigger for RA, especially in populations with a genetic predisposition [6]. Smoking may induce citrullination of peptide antigens present in the lungs, and the shared epitope alleles interact with smoking in the triggering of anti-citrulline immunity that may lead to ACPA-positive RA [7–9]. Two risk factors for RA, HLA-DRB1 shared epitope alleles and smoking, are also linked to adult periodontitis [10, 11]. Periodontitis is mainly induced by *Porphyromonas gingivalis* (*P. gingivalis*) infection, which, by subverting host immune defenses, leads to overgrowth of oral commensal bacteria causing inflammatory tissue destruction [12, 13]. This condition is characterized by the accumulation of large amounts of citrullinated proteins with similar patterns of hypercitrullination found in RA synovial fluid [14].

Since the 1980s, a number of studies have shown a possible association between RA and periodontitis, suggesting pathological similarities [15]. However, significant advances were not made until 1999, when it was found that *P. gingivalis* secretes a peptidylarginine deiminase (PAD)-like enzyme [16]. This was followed by a hypothesis by Rosenstein that periodontitis drives RA through the production of citrullinated antigens by *P. gingivalis* [17]. A periodontal pathogen, *P. gingivalis*, expresses an enzyme with PAD activity that mediates citrullination, in which arginine residues are deiminated to citrulline residues. This process may produce antibodies involved in the etiology of RA by breakdown of immunological tolerance to citrullinated antigens. To date, four citrullinated autoantigens have been defined: citrullinated fibrinogen, vimentin, collagen type II, and α-enolase [10, 11].

Although ACPAs, the autoantibodies directed against citrullinated peptides and proteins, are highly specific for RA, it should be noted that the enzyme-linked immunosorbent assay is based on synthetic cyclic citrullinated peptides (CCPs) and not equivalent to the detection of antibodies to citrullinated proteins *in vivo*. Currently, both smoking and *P. gingivalis* are plausible causative factors that warrant further investigation into the gene/environment/autoimmunity triad of RA etiology [18, 19].

1.2 Immunopathology of synovitis

The hallmark feature of arthritis in RA pathology is "synovitis," the inflammation of synovial membranes lining the inner surface of joint cavities, tendinous sheaths, and bursae. An autoimmune-mediated inflammatory response in joints leads to the formation of abnormal synovial tissue growth, the "rheumatoid pannus," which invades the joint space as well as adjacent components including bones and their protective layer of articular cartilage. The pathological milieu of the inflammatory synovial compartment, characterized by leukocyte infiltration comprising innate immune cells, e.g., monocytes, dendritic cells, mast cells, and innate lymphoid cells, as well as adaptive immune cells, e.g., Th1 and Th17 cells, B cells, plasmablasts, and plasma cells, is governed by a complex network of cytokines and chemokines. Dynamisation of this network leads to aggravation of the inflammatory response by activating endothelial cells and fibroblasts and ultimately triggering osteoclast generation through receptor activation of nuclear factor κ B ligand (RANKL) on T cells, B cells, and fibroblasts, with its receptor RANK on macrophages, dendritic cells, and preosteoblasts [20]. In the context of such inflammatory pathway, the key cytokines, i.e., tumor necrosis factor-α (TNF-α) and interleukin 6 (IL 6), play a critical role, as evidenced by therapeutic interventions targeting these factors resulting in remarkable clinical improvement in arthritis [21].

The recent work has shed light on a new scenario, in which the IL23/Th17 axis plays an essential role in bone loss, by favoring the generation of pathogenic ACPAs, via the secretion of IL-21 and IL-22, and by facilitating osteoclastogenesis, via the secretion of IL-17 [22]. As our understanding of molecular occurrence before the onset of RA has increased, it became evident that the interplay between mucosal events is relevant in the pathogenesis of the disease, in which oral and lung mucosa, under the stimuli of environmental factors, represents sites of ACPA production, while the intestinal dysbiosis increases the inflammatory state through increased Th17 polarization and IL-23/IL-17 axis activation (**Figure 1**) [23]. The recent discovery of the effect of ACPAs on osteoclastogenesis and on periarticular IL-8 production also suggests a mechanism that accounts for the transition from systemic autoimmunity to clinical manifestations [24].

1.3 Treatment of RA

Three decades ago, the treatment for RA was guided by a step-up approach, i.e., "the pyramid approach," in which nonsteroidal anti-inflammatory drugs (NSAIDs) and other conservative measures constituted first-line treatment, subsequently moving to more potent and cytotoxic drugs for persistent symptoms or progressive structural damage [25] (see **Figure 2**). This approach is no longer valid as RA has been recognized as causing substantial morbidity and mortality among those on the pyramid approach. Since then, RA treatment strategy has advanced dramatically. The routine administration of conventional disease-modifying antirheumatic drugs (cDMARDs), such as the anchor drug methotrexate, enabled physicians to ease RA symptoms with substantially better control of cartilage and bone erosion [26, 27] (**Table 1**).

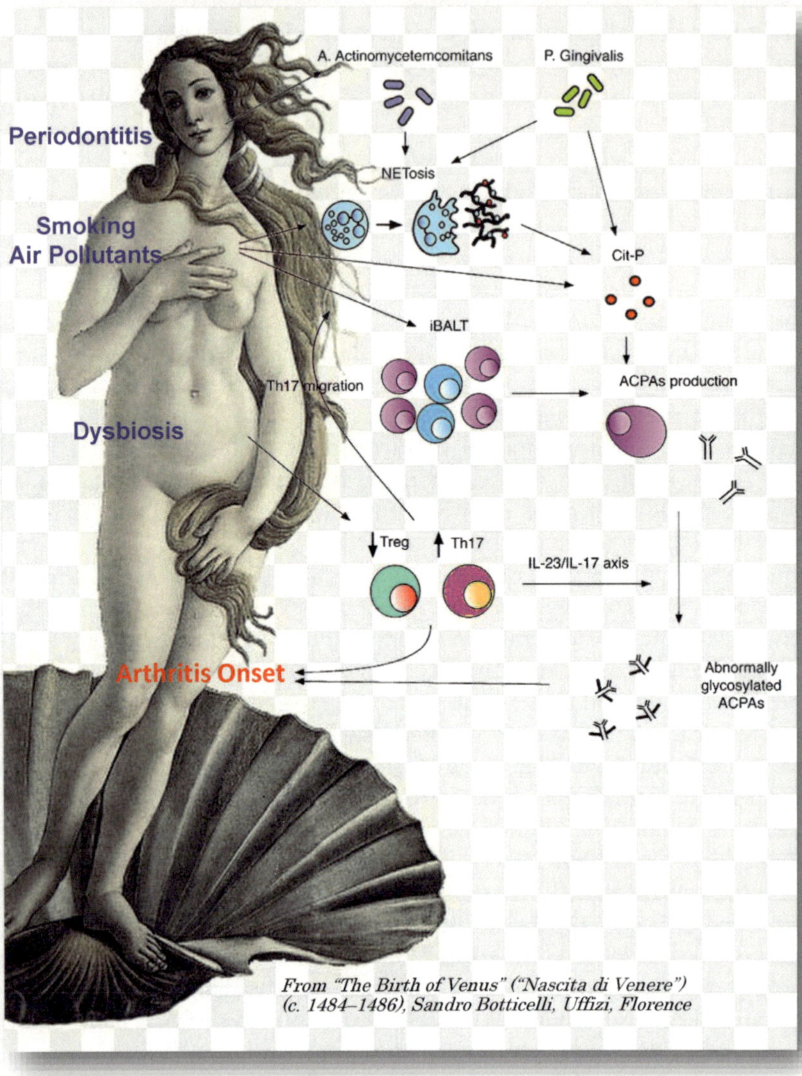

Figure 1.
Mucosa-environment interactions in the immuno-pathogenesis of RA. In the oral and lung mucosa, the stimuli of periodontal pathogens or environmental factors elicit production of citrullinated proteins, directly or through NETosis, and consequently result in ACPA production in subjects at risk. (1) At the periodontal level, Porphyromonas gingivalis (P. gingivalis) generates citrullinated peptides through PPAD. Moreover, through gingipains (Gp) (a family of proteases secreted by P. gingivalis), P. gingivalis increases Th17 polarization and induces NETosis. Aggregatibacter actinomycetemcomitans (A. actinomycetemcomitans) can also elicit the formation of citrullinated peptides, through the production of leukotoxin A (Lxt-A) and the induction of NETosis. Citrullinated peptides (Cit-P), recognized by specific B cells, induce ACPA production. (2) In the lung mucosa, smoke and air pollutants generate the formation of citrullinated antigens and NETosis. Mucosa reacts through the formation of iBALT (inducible bronchus associated lymphatic tissue) and elicits the local production of ACPAs, which can be detected in local secretions. (3) In systemic circulation, there is an increase of circulating Th17 and a reduction of Treg. T cells present an abnormal hypoglycolytic and hyperproliferative phenotype, and show an increased production of pro-inflammatory cytokines, such as IL-17. (4) In gut mucosa, dysbiosis of the intestinal microbiota inhibits the normal induction of Treg. Pathobiont species stimulate the activation of dendritic cells (DC), macrophages and innate lymphoid cells 3 (ILC3), leading to the polarization towards Th17, and the activation of the IL-23/IL-17 axis. Locally-produced Th17 can migrate through systemic circulation to other sites, inducing inflammation, abnormal Ig glycosylation, and iBALT formation. Specific B cells directed against luminal antigens can be activated in Peyer's patches or in local lymph nodes, migrating back in lamina propria where they produce secretory immunoglobulins (sIgs). Some of these B cells recognize antigens that cross-react with self-antigens via molecular mimicry. Finally, inflammatory cells and ACPAs lead to the onset of arthritis. Cit-p: citrullinated proteins; PPAD pathogen PAD; Gp: gingipains;*

Ltx-A: leukotoxin A; iBALT: inducible bronchus associated lymphatic tissue; sIgs: secretory immunoglobulins; ILC3: innate lymphoid cells 3; DC: dendritic cells; IL: interleukin.

**NETosis—the role in RA etiology: neutrophil extracellular traps (NETs) are chromatin-derived extracellular "spider's webs" that are expelled from neutrophils in response to infection or inflammatory stimuli. They were first described as an alternative defense mechanism by which neutrophils trap and kill microbes. NET-release represents a novel, unique form of cell death that is characterized by the discharge of decondensed chromatin and granular contents to the extracellular space, and is referred to as "NETosis", distinct from apoptosis and necrosis. Afterwards, it has become clear that NETs also render autoantigens in autoimmune diseases. NETs have been implicated in the development of autoimmunity in certain conditions such as RA and SLE through an exposure of externalized intracellular neoepitopes e.g., citrullinated peptides in RA and dsDNA and nuclear proteins in SLE. Currently, emerging evidence implicates NETs as a source of citrullinated neoepitopes in RA, causing loss of immune tolerance and development of autoantibodies to citrullinated proteins (ACPA). Citrulline residues in aggrecan and vimentin are preferentially recognized by antigen-presenting cells in individuals who carry the HLA-DRB1*04:01/04 allele, providing a molecular explanation for the strong association between this allele and the development of RA. Modified from Lucchino et al. [23].*

In addition, as the role of several key proinflammatory cytokines including TNF-α and IL-6, and cell-associated targets such as CD20 and co-stimulation molecules CD80/86, has been clarified, the treatment paradigm has changed with the advent of targeted biological therapies [28]. The emergence of a number of potent biological DMARDs (bDMARDs) has brought about a new therapeutic era that emphasizes the importance of early and aggressive treatment to prevent joint damage and induce remission [26, 29–32] (**Table 1**). It has become thoroughly evident that early suppression of disease activity is crucial. For instance, a large RA trial cohort study validated that early changes in MRI measures independently predicted X-ray and MRI progression, robustly suggesting the necessity of early intervention [33].

This conceptual trend in the treatment of RA was followed by new approval of the targeted synthetic DMARDs (tsDMARDs), such as small-molecule inhibitors of Janus kinase (JAK) enzymes [32, 34] (**Table 2**). The JAK family includes four members, JAK1, JAK2, JAK3, and tyrosine kinase 2 (TYK2). The different JAK isoforms, and the downstream signal transducer of activators of transcription

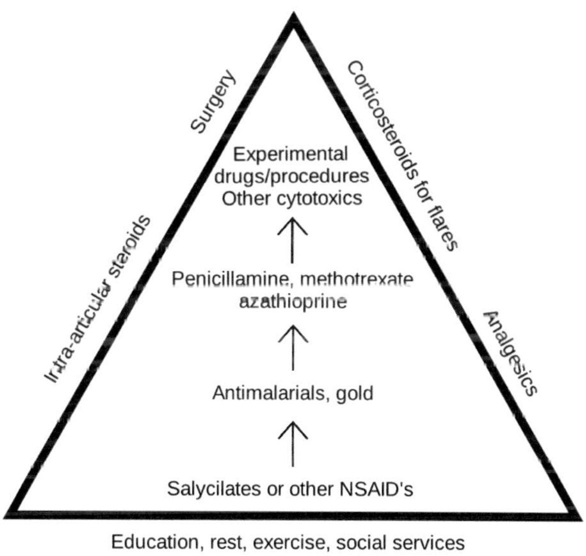

Figure 2.
The traditional treatment pyramid for RA, long since abandoned. Modified from Schumacher [62].

DMARD	Mechanism for rheumatoid arthritis	Adverse effects	Monthly cost[†]
Nonbiologic[*]			
More commonly used			
Methotrexate	Inhibits dihydrofolate reductase	Liver effects, teratogenesis, hair loss, oral ulcers	$
Leflunomide (Arava)	Inhibits pyrimidine synthesis	Liver effects, gastrointestinal effects, teratogenesis	$
Hydroxychloroquine (Plaquenil)	Antimalarial, blocks toll-like receptors	Rare ocular toxicity	$$
Sulfasalazine (Azulfidine)	Folate depletion, other mechanisms unknown	Anemia in G6PD deficiency, gastrointestinal effects	$
Minocycline (Minocin)	Antimicrobial, other mechanisms unknown	Drug-induced lupus erythematosus, *Clostridium difficile* colitis	$
Less commonly used			
Gold sodium thiomalate	Inhibits antigen processing, decreases cytokines (TNF, interleukin-6)	Skin, heme, renal effects	$$
Penicillamine (Cuprimine)	Chelates metal, other mechanisms unknown	Heme, renal effects	$$
Cyclophosphamide	Nitrogen mustard alkylating agent, cross-links DNA	Infertility, cancer, hemorrhagic cystitis	$$
Cyclosporine (Sandimmune)	Calcineurin inhibitor, decreases interleukin-2	Hypertension, renal effects, hirsutism	$$
Biologic[*]			
Anti-TNF agents			
Adalimumab (Humira)	Anti-TNF-α	TB, opportunistic infection	$$$
Certolizumab pegol (Cimzia)	Anti-TNF-α, pegylated	TB, opportunistic infection	$$$
Etanercept (Enbrel)	Anti-TNF-α, receptor	TB, opportunistic infection	$$$
Golimumab (Simponi)	Anti-TNF-α	TB, opportunistic infection	$$$
Infliximab (Remicade)	Anti-TNF-α	TB, opportunistic infection, infusion reaction	$$$
Other biologic agents			
Abatacept (Orencia)	Costimulator blocker, cytotoxic T lymphocyte antigen 4	Opportunistic infection	$$$
Anakinra (Kineret)	Anti-interleukin-1 receptor blocker	Opportunistic infection, injection site pain	$$$
Rituximab (Rituxan)	Anti-CD20, eliminates B cells	Infusion reaction, opportunistic infection, progressive multifocal leukoencephalopathy	$$$$
Tocilizumab (Actemra)	Anti-interleukin-6 receptor blocker	Opportunistic infection	$$$

G6PD = glucose-6-phosphate dehydrogenase; TB = tuberculosis; TNF = tumor necrosis factor.
Adapted from Wasserman [26].
[*]Nonbiologic drugs listed in approximate order of priority, biologic drugs listed in alphabetical order.
[†]$ = $30 to $100; $$ = $100 to $1000; $$$ = $1000 to $5000; $$$$ = more than $5000.

Table 1.
Biologic and nonbiologic DMARDs.

(STAT) proteins, are expressed in synovial tissue and cells [35]. The JAK–STAT pathway is currently thought to be an evolutionarily conserved signaling pathway engaged by diverse cytokines, interferons, growth factors, and hormones, providing a simple and elegant machinery whereby extracellular molecules regulate gene expression [36]. Each JAK family member selectively binds different receptor chains (**Figure 3**).

Many proinflammatory cytokines involved in RA pathogenesis bind to a specific group of type I and type II cytokine-receptors, which are structurally distinct from

Synthetic DMARDs
Conventional synthetic DMARDs
• Unknown target: methotrexate, sulfasalazine, chloroquine, hydroxychloroquine and gold salts • Known target: that is, dihydroorotate-dehydrogenase for leflunomide
Targeted synthetic DMARDs
• Janus kinase 1 (JAK1) and JAK2: baricitinib • JAK1, JAK2 and JAK3: tofacitinib
Biological DMARDs
Biological originator DMARDs
• Tumour necrosis factor: adalimumab, certolizumab, etanercept, golimumab and infliximab • IL-6 receptor: tocilizumab and sarilumab • IL-6: clazakizumab, olokizumab and sirukumab • CD80 and CD86 (involved in T cell co-stimulation): abatacept • CD20 (expressed by B cells): rituximab
Adapted from Smolen et al. [34].

Table 2.
Synthetic DMARDs and biologic DMARDs.

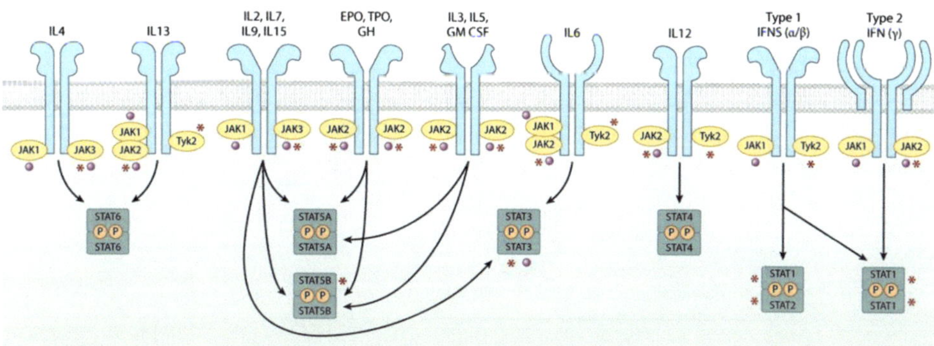

Figure 3.
*The JAK–STAT pathway. The four JAKs (JAK1, JAK2, JAK3, TYK2) are selectively bound to and therefore mediate signaling for various cytokine and hormone receptors. Different cytokines also have a propensity to activate certain STATs. Mutations in many of the gene encoding JAKs and STATs (indicated by an asterisk *) have been linked to human disease. A large number of medications targeting JAKs and, to a lesser degree, STATs (indicated by a ●) are being developed and used to treat human disease. Adapted from O'Shea et al. [36].*

other receptors such as those that bind TNF and IL-1. Since cytokines binding type I and II receptors are dependent on the JAK–STAT pathway for signal transduction, several JAK inhibitors ("jakinibs") with variable degrees of selectivity and specificity for the JAK enzymes have been tested in RA. Tofacitinib and baricitinib are the first orally available JAK inhibitors with selectivity for JAK 1 and 3 and JAK 1 and 2, respectively. Both have demonstrated rapid improvements in multiple outcome measures [37].

The latest 2019 update of the European League Against Rheumatism (EULAR) recommendations for the management of RA with synthetic and biological disease-modifying antirheumatic drugs provided consensus including the statement which elevated the JAK inhibitors ("tsDMARDs"), to the same recommendation level as bDMARDs [38]. The 2019 version of general overview of the RA management recommendations in form of an algorithm is depicted in **Figure 4** [32].

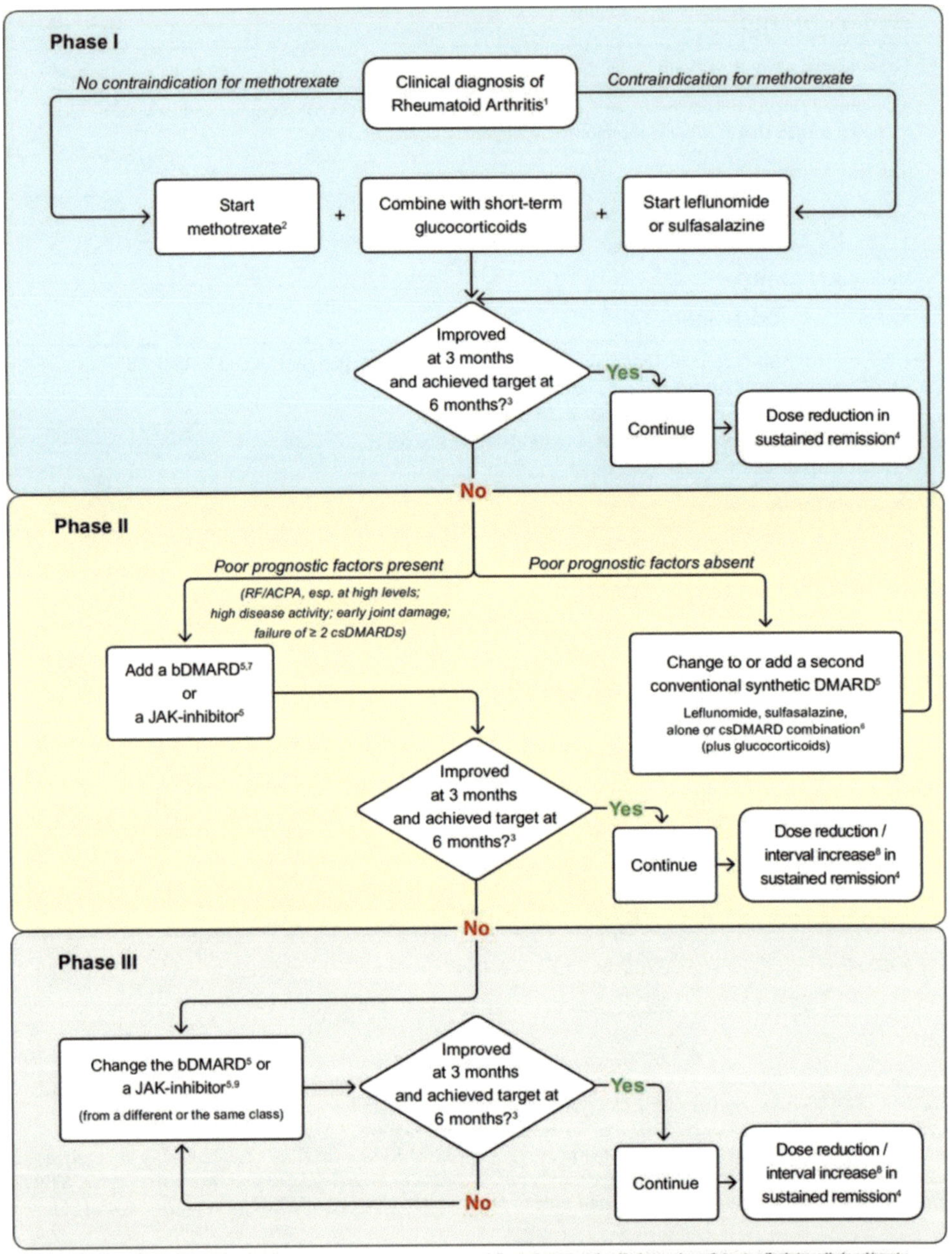

1. 2010 ACR-EULAR classification criteria can support early diagnosis.
2. "Methotrexate should be part of the first treatment strategy". While combination therapy of csDMARDs is not preferred by the Task Force, starting with methotrexate does not exclude its use in combination with other csDMARDs although more adverse events without added benefit are to be expected, especially if MTX is combined with glucocorticoids.
3. The treatment target is clinical remission according to ACR-EULAR definitions or, if remission is unlikely to be achievable, at least low disease activity; the target should be reached after 6 months, but therapy should be adapted or changed if insufficient improvement (less than 50% of disease activity) is seen after 3 months.
4. Sustained remission: ≥ 6 months ACR/EULAR index based or Boolean remission.
5. Consider contraindications and risks.
6. The most frequently used combination comprises methotrexate, sulfasalazine and hydroxychloroquine.
7. TNF-inhibitors (adalimumab, certolizumab, etanercept, golimumab, infliximab, including EMA/FDA approved bsDMARDs), abatacept, IL-6R inhibitors, or rituximab (under certain conditions); in patients who cannot use csDMARDs as comedication, IL6-inhibitors and tsDMARDs have some advantages.
8. Dose reduction or interval increase can be safely done with all bDMARDs and tsDMARDs with little risk of flares; stopping is associated with high flare rates; most but not all patients can recapture their good state upon re-institution of the same bDMARD/tsDMARD.
9. Efficacy and safety of bDMARDs after JAK-inhibitor failure is not fully known; also, efficacy and safety of an IL-6 pathway inhibitor after another one has failed is currently unknown. Efficacy and safety of a JAK-inhibitor after insufficient response to a previous JAK-inhibitor is unknown.

Figure 4.
Presentation of the 2019 update of the EULAR RA management recommendations in form of an algorithm. This is an abbreviated version aiming to provide a general overview, but it must be borne in mind that the algorithm cannot be separated from the details presented in the discussion of the individual recommendations in the paper which are part and parcel of these recommendations. ACPA, anti-citrullinated protein antibody; ACR, American College of Rheumatology; bDMARDs, biological DMARDs; bsDMARD, biosimilar DMARDs; csDMARDs, conventional synthetic DMARDs; DMARDs, disease-modifying antirheumatic drugs; EMA, European medicines agency; EULAR, European league against rheumatism; FDA, Food and Drug Administration; IL-6R, interleukin 6 receptor; JAK, Janus kinase; MTX, methotrexate; RA, rheumatoid arthritis; RF, rheumatoid factor; TNF, tumor necrosis factor; tsDMARDs, targeted synthetic DMARDs. Adapted from Smolen et al. [32].

1.4 Unmet diagnostic needs in RA

Given such revolutionary paradigm shift in the therapeutics for RA, it is warranted that we now readjust our focus towards innovative changes in the early diagnosis of RA. Today, physicians are required to diagnose RA earlier and with greater accuracy in order to start effective treatment as soon as possible and with greater confidence. Nonetheless, the reality in clinical practice is not simple at all. The diagnosis of RA continues to be mostly based on a combination of symptoms, signs, and results of investigations. However, because of the great variety of individual clinical presentations in RA, and since no single symptom or sign is specific for RA, accurate diagnosis may be hindered, especially in the early stages of disease when hallmark joint destruction may be absent or missed. Obviously, classification criteria for RA do exist, with a series of criteria having been created to define classic disease for clinical and both epidemiological studies. However, the application of classification criteria can give rise to both false-positive and false-negative classifications compared to the true clinical diagnosis [39]. In this context, we still do not have comprehensive diagnostic criteria of RA in the real clinical world.

Currently, among the clinically available imaging modalities, magnetic resonance imaging (MRI) is thought to be the most sensitive, and available evidence has led to its increasing use for assessing the active synovitis and bone damage central to many clinical RA studies including several of our previous reports [40–43].

Thus, to find a solution to the challenge of early diagnosis of RA, we aimed to develop practically useful diagnostic criteria which integrate gadolinium (Gd) contrast-enhanced magnetic resonance imaging (MRI) findings into clinical manifestations of the disease, which we will attempt to describe herein.

2. Attempts for accurate or earlier diagnosis of RA

2.1 The 1987 ACR classification criteria for RA: "old but gold" standard

As mentioned above, currently no validated diagnostic criteria exist for RA. By contrast, a few sets of classification criteria have been developed and modified over time. Classification criteria are standardized definitions that are primarily aimed to collect homogenous cohorts of patients with typical disease, primarily for clinical and epidemiological studies [44]. Although they are not intended to capture the entire universe of patients with the disease, they may provide some framework to support diagnosis and are often used in this way in daily practice.

The most historically notable classification criteria which have been used in RA are the American College of Rheumatology (ACR) criteria revised in 1987 by the American Rheumatism Association, published by Arnett et al. [45] (**Table 3**). At the time the 1987 criteria were presented, sensitivity and specificity were reported to be 91–94% and 89%, respectively. They have been widely applied for diagnosis, as well. However, the 1987 criteria, which were developed based on established patients with an average disease duration of 7.7 years, have come to be recognized as having poor performance for diagnosing early RA. A systemic literature review by Banal et al. of 138 publications comprising 7438 patients (including 3883 cases of RA) reported that the sensitivity and specificity of the 1987 criteria (in the list format) for early RA (<1 year) were 77% (68–84%) and 77% (68–84%), respectively, compared to 79% (71–85%) and 90% (84–94%), respectively, for established RA (>1 year) [46]. The Norfolk Arthritis Register report by Harrison et al. demonstrated that only 50% of RA patients fulfilled the 1987 criteria at 6 months and only

Criterion	Description
Morning stiffness	Morning stiffness in and around the joints that lasts at least 1 hour before maximal improvement
Arthritis in three or more areas	At least three joint areas that simultaneously have soft-tissue swelling or fluid (not bone overgrowth alone) observed by a physician (the 14 possible joint areas are the right and left PIP, MCP, wrist, elbow, knee, ankle, and MTP joints)
Arthritis of hand joints	At least one of the following joint areas is swollen: wrist, MCP, or PIP joint (see description of second criterion)
Symmetric arthritis	Simultaneous involvement of the same joint areas listed for the second criterion on both sides of the body (bilateral involvement of PIP, MCP, or MTP joints is acceptable without absolute symmetry)
Rheumatoid nodules	Subcutaneous nodules over bone prominences or extensor surfaces or in juxtaarticular regions observed by a physician
Serum rheumatoid factor	Demonstration of abnormal amounts of serum rheumatoid factor with any method that has yielded positive results in <5% of healthy control subjects
Radiographic changes	Changes typical of rheumatoid arthritis on posteroanterior radiographs of the hand and wrist; these must include erosions or unequivocal bone decalcification localized to or most marked adjacent to the involved joints (osteoarthritic changes alone do not qualify)

Note: For classification purposes, a patient is said to have rheumatoid arthritis if he or she has satisfied at least four of the seven criteria. The first four criteria must be present for at least 6 weeks. Patients with two clinical diagnoses are not excluded. MCP = metacarpophalangeal, MTP = metatarsophalangeal, PIP = proximal interphalangeal. Adapted from Arnett et al. [45].

Table 3.
The ACR 1987 revised criteria for the classification of rheumatoid arthritis.

80% even at 2 years after enrolment [47]. Thus, the 1987 criteria do not appear to be well-suited as a diagnostic measure of short-duration RA. Emerging evidence on the response of arthritis to early intervention with DMARDs indicates the existence of "a window of opportunity in RA," a time during which aggressive treatment accounts for long-term benefits in outcome. Therefore, to meet clinical needs, better diagnostic measures are required to identify RA patients at the earliest stages of the disease.

2.2 The 2010 ACR/EULAR classification criteria for RA

Since 2007, the ACR and EULAR have been working collaboratively to create new classification criteria for RA, which were finally published in 2010 [48] (**Table 4**). The 2010 criteria are an effort to facilitate earlier diagnosis of RA in patients who may not meet the 1987 ACR criteria. For example, they do not include the presence of rheumatoid nodules or radiographic erosive changes, both of which are less likely in early RA. The 2010 criteria consist of a classification scoring system, laying emphasis on small joint involvement as well rheumatoid factor (RF) or ACPA seropositivity. It should be noted that RF is not specific for RA and can be detected in patients with other disorders, such as viral hepatitis C, and in healthy elderly individuals [49, 50] (**Table 5**). Although ACPA is more specific for RA, it may be present in other rheumatic diseases and some infectious diseases [51] (**Table 6**). We know approximately 50–80% of patients with RA have RF, ACPA, or both [52]. Acute-phase reactants such as C-reactive protein and erythrocyte sedimentation rate are also part of the criteria. As shown in **Table 4**, in the new classification criteria, the definition of RA requires at least a single clinically swollen joint for inclusion entry and the absence

	Score
Target population (Who should be tested?): Patients who	
1. have at least 1 joint with definite clinical synovitis (swelling)* 2. with the synovitis not better explained by another disease†	
Classification criteria for RA (score-based algorithm: add score of categories A–D; a score of ≥6/10 is needed for classification of a patient as having definite RA)‡	
A. Joint involvement§	
1 large joint¶	0
2–10 large joints	1
1–3 small joints (with or without involvement of large joints)#	2
4–10 small joints (with or without involvement of large joints)	3
>10 joints (at least 1 small joint)**	5
B. Serology (at least 1 test result is needed for classification)††	
Negative RF *and* negative ACPA	0
Low-positive RF *or* low-positive ACPA	2
High-positive RF *or* high-positive ACPA	3
C. Acute-phase reactants (at least 1 test result is needed for classification)‡‡	
Normal CRP *and* normal ESR	0
Abnormal CRP *or* abnormal ESR	1
D. Duration of symptoms§§	
<6 weeks	0
≥6 weeks	1

**The criteria are aimed at classification of newly presenting patients. In addition, patients with erosive disease typical of rheumatoid arthritis (RA) with a history compatible with prior fulfillment of the 2010 criteria should be classified as having RA. Patients with longstanding disease, including those whose disease is inactive (with or without treatment) who, based on retrospectively available data, have previously fulfilled the 2010 criteria should be classified as having RA.*
†Differential diagnoses vary among patients with different presentations, but may include conditions such as systemic lupus erythematosus, psoriatic arthritis, and gout. If it is unclear about the relevant differential diagnoses to consider, an expert rheumatologist should be consulted.
‡Although patients with a score of <6/10 are not classifiable as having RA, their status can be reassessed and the criteria might be fulfilled cumulatively over time.
§Joint involvement refers to any swollen *or* tender *joint on examination, which may be confirmed by imaging evidence of synovitis. Distal interphalangeal joints, first carpometacarpal joints, and first metatarsophalangeal joints are* excluded from assessment*. Categories of joint distribution are classified according to the location and number of involved joints, with placement into the highest category possible based on the pattern of joint involvement.*
¶"Large joints" refers to shoulders, elbows, hips, knees, and ankles.
#"Small joints" refers to the metacarpophalangeal joints, proximal interphalangeal joints, second through fifth metatarsophalangeal joints, thumb interphalangeal joints, and wrists.
***In this category, at least 1 of the involved joints must be a small joint; the other joints can include any combination of large and additional small joints, as well as other joints not specifically listed elsewhere (e.g., temporomandibular, acromioclavicular, sternoclavicular, etc.).*
††Negative refers to IU values that are less than or equal to the upper limit of normal (ULN) for the laboratory and assay; low-positive refers to IU values that are higher than the ULN but ≤3 times the ULN for the laboratory and assay; high-positive refers to IU values that are >3 times the ULN for the laboratory and assay. Where rheumatoid factor (RF) information is only available as positive or negative, a positive result should be scored as low-positive for RF. ACPA = anti–citrullinated protein antibody.
‡‡Normal/abnormal is determined by local laboratory standards. CRP = C-reactive protein; ESR = erythrocyte sedimentation rate.
§§Duration of symptoms refers to patient self-report of the duration of signs or symptoms of synovitis (e.g., pain, swelling, tenderness) of joints that are clinically involved at the time of assessment, regardless of treatment status.
Adapted from Aletaha et al. [48].

Table 4.
The 2010 ACR/EULAR classification criteria for rheumatoid arthritis.

of other diseases (alternative diagnoses) better explaining the clinical symptoms. Thereafter, the classification is based on a total score from individual items in four domains including the number of involved joints, serological abnormalities, elevated acute-phase reactants, and duration of symptoms.

Disease	RF frequency, %
Arthritis	
Rheumatoid arthritis	70–90
Juvenile idiopathic arthritis	5
Psoriatic arthritis	<15
Reactive arthritis	<5
Other connective tissue diseases	
Primary Sjögren's syndrome	75–95
Mixed connective tissue disease	50–60
Systemic lupus erythematosus	15–35
Systemic sclerosis	20–30
Dermatomyositis/polymyositis	20
Systemic vasculitides	5–20
Infectious diseases	
Bacterial infections	
Subacute bacterial endocarditis	40
Chlamydia pneumoniae infection	
Klebsiella pneumoniae infection	
Syphilis primary-tertiary	8–37
Tuberculosis	15
Viral infections	
Coxsackie B virus infection	15
Dengue virus infection	10
EBV and CMV infections	20
Hepatitis A, B and C virus infection	25
HCV infection	40–76
Herpes virus infection	10–15
HIV infection	10–20
Measles	8–15
Parvovirus infection	10
Rubella	15
Parasitic	
Chagas	15–25
Malaria	15–18
Onchocerciasis	10
Toxoplasmosis	10–12
Other diseases	
Mixed cryoglobulinemia type II	100*
Liver cirrhosis	25
Primary biliary cirrhosis	45–70
Malignancy	5–25
After multiple immunizations	10–15
Chronic sarcoidosis	5–30
Healthy individuals	
Healthy 50-year olds	5
Healthy 70-year olds	10–25

**Monoclonal IgM rheumatoid factors.*
RF: rheumatoid factor; CMV: cytomegalovirus; EBV: Epstein-Barr virus; HCV: hepatitis C virus; HIV: human immunodeficiency virus.
Adapted from Ingegnoli et al. [50].

Table 5.
Rheumatoid factor frequency in different diseases and conditions.

The primary aim of creating the 2010 criteria was described as not for developing diagnostic criteria but rather to facilitate the study of patients with earlier stages of RA. However, they have become widely used as an aid in the diagnosis of RA in

	N	ACPA* positive, no. (%)
Psoriatic arthritis	1343	115 (8.6)
Systemic lupus erythematosus	1078	84 (7.8)
Sjögren's syndrome	609	35 (5.7)
Spondylarthropathy	431	10 (2.3)
Scleroderma/CREST syndrome	380	26 (6.8)
Hepatitis C/cryoglobulinemia	285	10 (3.5)
Osteoarthritis	182	4 (2.2)
Hepatitis B	176	1 (0.6)
Juvenile idiopathic arthritis	169	13 (7.7)
Polymyalgia rheumatica	146	0 (0)
Vasculitis/Wegener's granulomatosis	107	5 (4.7)
Tuberculosis	96	33 (34.3)
Polymyositis/dermatomyositis	75	0 (0)
Fibromyalgia	74	2 (2.7)
Gout and pseudogout	58	0 (0)

**ACPA = anti-citrullinated peptide antibody; CREST = calcinosis, Raynaud's phenomenon, esophageal dysmotility, sclerodactyly, telangiectasias syndrome.*
Adapted from Aggarwal et al. [51].

Table 6.
Detection of ACPAs in diseases other than rheumatoid arthritis.

clinical practice, resulting in helping clinicians and researchers to become aware of the 2010 criteria's strengths and limitations as well. First of all, regarding entry criterion of the target population, the sentence "patients who with the synovitis not better explained by another disease" is quite tricky. Annotation states that "Differential diagnoses differ in patients with different presentations, but may include conditions such as systemic lupus erythematosus, psoriatic arthritis, and gout. If it is unclear about the relevant differential diagnosis to consider, an expert rheumatologist should be consulted." Most rheumatologists know that there are many mimicking conditions to be distinguished from RA. The easy "ask-the-expert" attitude may be paradoxical to the principle of having criteria. Furthermore, Kaneko et al. identified a problem with the scoring criteria, which weigh relatively heavily in favor of serology, reporting a sensitivity as low as 15.8% when both RF and ACPA are negative. For instance, a seronegative person having 10 swollen joints for >6 weeks, with elevated CRP and ESR and destructive joint disease, would not achieve a total score of 6 per the new criteria [53]. Thus, several limitations of the 2010 criteria have already been recognized which hinder their use in daily practice.

3. Notion of early RA

Since early diagnosis and treatment with newly developed antirheumatic drugs including bDMARDs and tsDMARDs have been advocated for patients with RA, the understanding of "early" RA has changed. Formerly, early RA denoted disease of less than 2 years, or used to be sometimes less than 12 months duration. However, today, many rheumatologists may even see patients with symptom duration of less than 6 weeks. While the definition of early RA is still heterogeneous, two-thirds of rheumatologists use the term "early" for symptoms shorter than 3 months. Currently, in general, early RA patients are preferentially regarded as those with symptoms of less than 3 months duration [54].

Besides the notion of disease duration, clinical practice informs us that there are a number of existing clinical factors which may also suggest early RA. These may include persistent pain in multiple joints despite normal joint radiography without fulfillment of RA classification criteria. Similarly, because clinicians may care for RA patient longitudinally over time, they are more likely to appreciate early manifestations, even in hindsight, as exemplified by the following common clinical situations:

1. Patients in the early stage of RA may not manifest soft tissue swelling (arthritis) of three or more joints as described in the 1987 classification criteria.

2. Patients in the early stage of RA may not necessarily present with unequivocally symmetric swelling (arthritis).

3. Patients in the very early stage of RA may not demonstrate serological abnormalities such as elevated acute-phase reactants during which time CRP and ESR are often unremarkable.

4. Inclusion of the presence of autoantibodies as major criteria for diagnosis may not be fair, considering that a significant proportion of patients are seronegative. As evidence suggests that seronegative RA represents a disease entity clinically and immunogenetically distinct from seropositive RA, it may well be inappropriate to apply RF to a mixed population of seropositive and seronegative patients [55].

5. Almost all RA patients have joint symptoms in the hands; even though the knee, ankle, or foot joint symptoms may precede hand pain, most patients have some joint pain of the hands at the time of presentation.

On the basis of these fundamental understandings, we aimed to develop practically useful criteria for the early diagnosis of RA by integrating Gd contrast-enhanced MRI findings with clinical manifestations of the disease.

4. Benefits of MRI in diagnosing RA

Radiographs are the current gold standard for evaluating joint damage in RA, and it is likely that radiography will continue to be used in daily clinical practice for monitoring arthritis disease progression. However, conventional radiography is not sensitive enough for depicting bone damage in early disease and is also insufficient for assessing synovial inflammation. These limitations have led to emerging interest in the multiplanar imaging abilities of MRI in RA and to wider use of MRI for assessing synovitis and bone damage [56].

4.1 Basic principles of MRI and RA pathology on MRI

The principles of MRI are briefly explained here. Upon being placed in external magnetic fields, hydrogen protons in human tissue align. They acquire energy (resonance) when excited by an external electro-magnetic pulse at a characteristic resonance frequency, with a consequent decrease in longitudinal magnetization and increase in transverse magnetization. When the pulse is turned off, protons return to their previous low-energy state. The net movement of hydrogen protons elicits an electric current that is measured as the MR signal [57]. The presentation of particular tissues depends on their hydrogen proton content. In common MRI sequences, a T1-weighted (T1W) image represents fat-containing tissues, for example, the high signal of the bone marrow. By contrast, on T2W images, not only fat but fluid demonstrates high signal. The available techniques of fat suppression eliminate high signal from fat, consequently making fluid and inflammation better evident.

MRI can be used to assess inflammation (synovitis and bone edema) and damage (bone erosion) in the joint. Synovitis is depicted as an area in the synovial compartment that shows enhancement (signal intensity increase) on T1-weighted images after venous injection of gadolinium contrast. MRI bone erosion is visualized as a sharply marginated bone lesion, with correct juxta-articular localization and typical signal characteristics, i.e., loss of normal low-signal intensity of the cortical bone and loss of normal high-signal intensity of the trabecular bone on T1-weighted images. MRI bone edema is visualized as a lesion within the trabecular bone, with ill-defined margins and signal characteristics consistent with increased water content, i.e., high-signal intensity on T2-weighted fat-saturated and STIR images and low-signal intensity on T1-weighted images. Bone edema may occur alone or surrounding an area of erosion or other bone abnormality. Outcome Measures in Rheumatology (OMERACT), an independent initiative of international health professionals serving for the validation of clinical and radiographic outcome measures, has iteratively developed an RA-MRI scoring system (RAMRIS) framework for the evaluation of inflammatory and destructive changes in RA hands (metacarpophalangeal, MCP, joints) and wrists (carpal bones, distal radius, distal ulna, metacarpal bases) [58].

4.2 MRI of synovitis

Since synovitis is the earliest abnormality to occur in RA, MR imaging of synovitis is currently the best way to identify the earliest changes critical for early diagnosis of RA. MRI signatures of synovitis include increased synovial volume, increased water content, and contrast enhancement, i.e., increased signal intensity after intravenous injection of contrast material.

Synovitis reveals intermediate-to-low-signal intensity on T1-weighted images, whereas due to the increased water content of synovitis, various signal intensities can be viewed on T2-weighted images including the high signal of hypervascular synovium, as well as the low-signal characteristic of fibrosis.

The use of intravenous Gd-based contrast material plays an important role in MRI identification of synovitis. A number of dynamic MRI studies have demonstrated a good correlation between MRI synovium volume estimates and arthroscopic and histological inflammation scores [59]. The most used contrast material for evaluating synovitis is the paramagnetic agent, gadolinium-diethylenetriamine penta-acid (Gd-DTPA). This agent shortens the relaxation time of adjacent tissues, thereby improving the contrast between tissues on imaging. Uptake of Gd-DTPA depends upon vascularity and capillary permeability of tissues, making it particularly useful in visualizing sites of inflammation.

Contrast-enhanced T1-weighted images are sensitive and specific in the assessment of acute synovitis. After intravenous administration of Gd-DTPA, acute synovitis enhances rapidly and intensely, unlike joint effusion, which does not enhance in the early phase. Early-phase enhancement lasts for approximately 5 min after contrast injection [60]. Since gadolinium may diffuse into the synovial joint fluid, images acquired more than 10 min after injection may not accurately depict the extent of synovitis. In contrast, joint fluid enhancement appears within minutes

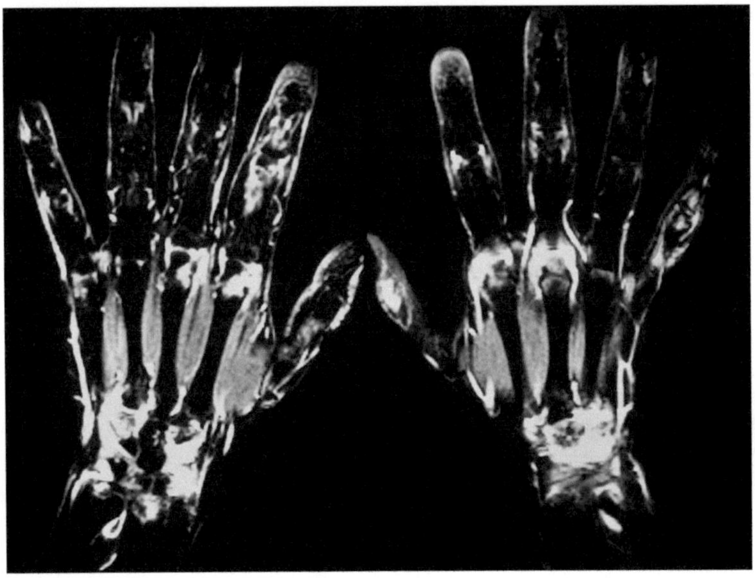

Figure 5.
MR imaging signs of synovitis in our study. Fat-suppressed contrast-enhanced T1-weighted coronal MR imaging from the volar aspect of the hand in a patient with early RA, in whom radiographic assessment was normal. There is marked synovial enhancement at the joints of PIP, MCP, as well as wrist joints.

and reaches a plateau after 30 min. The use of fat suppression increases visual contrast between the inflamed synovium and adjacent structures on contrast-enhanced T1-weighted images [61]. OMERACT defines synovitis as an area in the synovial compartment with increased contrast enhancement whose thickness exceeds the width of normal synovium [58]. For the evaluation of synovitis in early RA, we used coronal Gd-enhanced fat-suppressed T1-weighted MR images from both hands. The hand was chosen for MRI assessment given that is the most clinically affected area in RA. **Figure 5** represents fat-suppressed contrast-enhanced MRI from the volar aspect of the hand in a patient with early RA in our study, in whom radiographic assessment was normal. Remarkable synovial enhancement at the PIP, MCP, as well as wrist joints is noted.

5. Approach to the formulation of diagnostic criteria for early RA

5.1 Characteristics of contrast-enhanced MRI in active RA

First of all, we need to properly incorporate clinically significant MRI findings into our diagnostic criteria for early RA. Therefore, at the outset, preliminary studies of Gd-enhanced MRI were conducted to distinguish characteristics of synovial MR images in active RA, using 20 patients with definitive clinical diagnoses of RA (17 women, 3 men, ages 21–72 years, mean age 47.8 years), consisting of 17 active cases and 3 inactive cases in remission [40–43].

The MR imaging protocol we used is as follows: MR imaging of the hand was performed with a 1.5-Tesla superconducting magnet (MRT 200 FX/II, Toshiba) equipped with a circular surface coil 20 cm in diameter. Multiple coronal MR images of the hand were obtained using a fat-suppressed T1-weighted spin-echo sequence (repetition time msec/echo time msec = 380/20, 4 mm section thickness with 1 mm intersection gap). Contrast-enhanced images were obtained after bolus injection of 0.1 mmol/kg gadopentetate dimeglumine (Magnevist, Schering) into a vein in the arm. MR images were acquired within 5 min after injection to avoid diffusion of the contrast material into joints.

As a result, we found bilateral enhancement in the wrist joints (carpal bones, distal radius, distal ulna, metacarpal bases) in 17 cases of active RA and the metacarpophalangeal (MCP) or proximal interphalangeal (PIP) joints in 14 cases. By contrast, no enhancement was seen in any of the three inactive cases in remission. On the basis of these convincing results, we decided to focus on the bilateral enhancement of the synovia in the PIP, MCP, or wrist joints, which may best characterize the MRI findings of synovitis associated with active RA.

Thus, we established our preliminary criteria for the diagnosis of early RA using MR imaging. These preliminary criteria were comprised of two steps with the first requiring clinical findings suggestive of RA, including polyarthralgia of hands in three joints or more ("entry criteria"). The second step involved MRI findings indicating bilateral synovial enhancement seen in any PIP, MCP, or wrist joints on Gd-enhanced MRI ("MRI criteria"). Bilateral involvement of PIP, MCP, or wrist joints is acceptable though absolute symmetry is not required. RA was defined by fulfilling the both entry criteria and MRI criteria.

To evaluate the performance of these preliminary criteria, we conducted a provisional study to investigate the difference between the early RA and the other conditions than RA in Gd-MRI findings. We selected patients with early RA, defined as those carrying a definitive clinical diagnosis of RA made by a board-certified, trained rheumatologist, but without having radiographic changes. Sixteen patients (15 women, 1 man, aged 19–76 years, mean age 49.9 years) with early RA and 11 non-RA controls (9 women, 2 men, 19–52 years, mean age 41.7 years), who fulfilled the entry criteria, were enrolled. Non-RA controls consisted of patients with systemic lupus erythematosus (2 cases), Sjögren's syndrome (one case), Behçet's disease (one case), palindromic rheumatoid arthritis (one case), reactive arthritis (two cases), viral arthritis (one case), and nonspecific transient self-limiting arthritis (three cases). We evaluated the performance of the preliminary criteria among cases that fulfilled entry criteria, including sensitivity and specificity analyses. Our preliminary MRI criteria showed 100% sensitivity, 73% specificity, and 89% accuracy in differentiating RA from other conditions.

Since that study, from daily experience using contrast-enhanced MRI in a large number of clinical cases, we have found that enhancement in the synovium may also be observed occasionally in patients with systemic lupus erythematosus, dermatomyositis, polymyositis, mixed connective tissue disease, and Behçet's disease.

5.2 Proposed "diagnostic criteria for early RA with MRI findings"

On the basis of our preliminary studies, we created provisional criteria under the title "diagnostic criteria for early RA with MRI findings" (**Table** 7).

These provisional diagnostic criteria comprise two domains. The first domain consists of clinical findings suggestive of RA and includes entry criteria requiring polyarthralgia of hands (joint pain of three or more joint areas confirmed by a physician) and exclusion criteria that exclude other rheumatic conditions, i.e., systemic lupus erythematosus (SLE), dermatomyositis and polymyositis (PM/DM), mixed connective tissue disease (MCTD), primary Sjögren's syndrome (SS), and Behçet's disease (BD). The second domain constitutes the MRI criteria, requiring Gd-enhanced MRI findings indicating bilateral synovial enhancement seen in any PIP, MCP, or wrist joints. Bilateral involvement of PIP, MCP, or carpal joints of wrists is acceptable, and absolute symmetry is not required to meet the domain criteria. Early RA is defined by fulfilling all conditions of both domains.

Diagnosis of RA is defined by fulfilling all conditions of following both domains
Clinical domain—clinical findings suggestive of RA: 1. **Entry criteria:** presence of polyarthralgia in hands (three or more joint areas) 2. **Exclusion criteria:** exclusion of other rheumatic conditions, i.e., **systemic lupus erythematosus (SLE),** **dermatomyositis and polymyositis (PM/DM),** **mixed connective tissue disease (MCTD),** **primary Sjögren's syndrome (SS), and** **Behçet's disease (BD)** • **If case meets entry criteria and does not meet any exclusion criteria, proceed to MRI criteria**
MRI domain—MRI findings suggestive of RA: 3. **MRI criteria:** bilateral synovial enhancement on Gd-enhanced MRI* **in the proximal interphalangeal (PIP), or** **metacarpophalangeal (MCP), or** **wrist joints**

**Symmetrical involvement in bilateral joints not required.*

Table 7.
The diagnostic criteria for early RA with MRI findings (proposal).

5.3 Validation of "diagnostic criteria for early RA with MRI findings" in prospective study

We evaluated our provisional diagnostic criteria for early rheumatoid arthritis with MRI findings in a prospective study, approved by our institutional review board. The validity of the diagnostic criteria was assessed by acquisition of final diagnoses at the end of the clinical follow-up of a certain duration. Final diagnoses were made comprehensively. Subjects included patients presenting with polyarthralgia who visited rheumatology clinic at our institution. At the end of recruitment, we enrolled 50 consecutive patients including 9 men and 41 women (mean age, 44 years; range, 19–74 years old). All enrollees met entry criteria defined as the presence of polyarthralgia in hands in three or more joint areas. The diagnosis of RA or non-RA was made after careful clinical follow-up by trained rheumatologists. The final diagnosis of RA was established according to physical

Subjects: 50 cases (41 women and 9 men, average age = 44 years old)
Observation period: mean duration = 776 days
Drop out: two cases

Final diagnoses:

Disease category	**n**
RA	**26**
Non-RA	**22**
Arthritis related to viral infection	3
Sjögren's syndrome	2*
Osteoarthritis	4
Reactive arthritis	1
Cryoglobulinemia	1
Palindromic rheumatism	1
Unclassified self-limited arthritis	10

**Primary Sjögren's syndrome diagnosed during the study period.*

Table 8.
Demographic profiles of patients with RA and non-RA diseases.

	No. of patients		True positive	True negative	False positive	False negative	Sensitivity (%)	Specificity (%)	Accuracy
Final Dx	**RA**	**Non-RA**							
	26	22							
Proposed criteria	28	20	25	19*	3**	1	96%	86%	92%
ACR 1987 criteria	19	29	18	21	1	8	69%	95%	81%

**Predictive value of negative results: 95%.*
***False positive: cryoglobulinemia = 1; arthritis related to viral infection = 1, osteoarthritis = 1.*

Table 9.
Sensitivity, specificity, and accuracy of proposed criteria for rheumatoid arthritis.

findings compatible with RA or radiographic changes specific for RA and after ruling out other disease conditions. The average duration of follow-up from first visit was 776 days (range, 117–2161 days). Two of the 50 enrolled patients were lost to follow-up prior to diagnosis, and subsequent medical information was not available; they were excluded from the analysis.

After a thorough follow-up period of careful clinical observation, a final pool of 48 patients had confirmed diagnoses: 26 patients had RA, and 22 had non-RA conditions. Patient disease profiles are shown in **Table 8**. Statistics of diagnostic performance is presented in **Table 9**. The proposed diagnostic criteria for early RA with MRI findings was able to diagnose 25 of 26 patients with RA with high accuracy. False positives occurred in three patients, yielding a sensitivity of 96%, specificity of 86%, and accuracy of 92%, indicating high diagnostic performance. In particular, it should be noted that the criteria effectively ruled out RA with a high negative predictive value of 95%.

Thus, our study objectively demonstrated that the "diagnostic criteria of early rheumatoid arthritis with MRI findings" was clinically quite effective in making early diagnoses of RA, though there is a need to validate the criteria with a larger sample of patients.

6. Conclusions

The combined use of MRI measures and clinical findings for the diagnosis of early RA holds considerable promise for improving the accuracy of early diagnosis of RA and may be effective in facilitating earlier use of interventions for this progressive disease.

The increasing use of MRI for the diagnosis of RA may come at cost, and therefore inappropriate use and overuse should be avoided. Nonetheless, MRI provides a great advantage over conventional radiography in terms of quantitatively identifying inflamed synovium tissues with a high degree of sensitivity. The incorporation of MRI findings together with clinical findings into the criteria for the diagnosis of early RA demonstrates excellent diagnostic performance.

Early and accurate diagnosis, which can be achieved through the introduction of our proposed criteria, can prevent prolonged anxiety and suffering in RA patients who live with persistent joint pain and disability. Furthermore, early diagnosis may lead to a number of social benefits including enabling patients an earlier return to work and to active lives through early treatment.

We believe our novel diagnostic criteria for early RA integrated with MRI findings will contribute substantially to daily clinical practice as well as to the epidemiology and basic science of RA.

Disclosure statement

The authors have declared no conflicts of interest.

Patient consent

The authors have declared in the published articles that the informed consent was obtained from the patients.

Ethical approval

The authors have declared in the published articles that the protocols were approved by the institutional review board.

Author details

Akira Takeda[1]* and Hideharu Sugimoto[2]

1 Division of Clinical Immunology and Rheumatology, International University of Health and Welfare Hospital, Nasu-Shiobara, Tochigi, Japan

2 Department of Radiology, School of Medicine, Jichi Medical University, Shimotsuke, Tochigi, Japan

*Address all correspondence to: akitake@iuhw.ac.jp

References

[1] Huizinga TW, Amos CI, van der Helm-van Mil AH, Chen W, van Gaalen FA, Jawaheer D, et al. Refining the complex rheumatoid arthritis phenotype based on specificity of the HLA-DRB1 shared epitope for antibodies to citrullinated proteins. Arthritis and Rheumatism. 2005;**52**(11): 3433-3438

[2] Scally SW, Petersen J, Law SC, Dudek NL, Nel HJ, Loh KL, et al. A molecular basis for the association of the HLA-DRB1 locus, citrullination, and rheumatoid arthritis. Journal of Experimental Medicine. 2013;**210**(12): 2569-2582. DOI: 10.1084/jem.20131241

[3] Wordsworth BP, Lanchbury JS, Sakkas LI, Welsh KI, Panayi GS, Bell JI. HLA-DR4 subtype frequencies in rheumatoid arthritis indicate that DRB1 is the major susceptibility locus within the HLA class II region. Proceedings of the National Academy of Sciences of the United States of America. 1989;**86**(24): 10049-10053. DOI: 10.1073/pnas.86.24.10049

[4] Viatte S, Plant D, Raychaudhuri S. Genetics and epigenetics of rheumatoid arthritis. Nature Reviews Rheumatology. 2013;**9**(3):141-153. DOI: 10.1038/nrrheum.2012.237

[5] Sugiyama D, Nishimura K, Tamaki K, Tsuji G, Nakazawa T, Morinobu A, et al. Impact of smoking as a risk factor for developing rheumatoid arthritis: A meta-analysis of observational studies. Annals of the Rheumatic Diseases. 2010;**69**(1):70-81. DOI: 10.1136/ard.2008.096487

[6] Redlich K, Hayer S, Ricci R, David JP, Tohidast-Akrad M, Kollias G, et al. Osteoclasts are essential for TNF-alpha-mediated joint destruction. The Journal of Clinical Investigation. 2002;**110**(10): 1419-1427

[7] Makrygiannakis D, Hermansson M, Ulfgren AK, Nicholas AP, Zendman AJ, Eklund A, et al. Smoking increases peptidylarginine deiminase 2 enzyme expression in human lungs and increases citrullination in BAL cells. Annals of the Rheumatic Diseases. 2008; **67**(10):1488-1492. DOI: 10.1136/ard.2007.075192

[8] Padyukov L, Silva C, Stolt P, Alfredsson L, Klareskog L. A gene-environment interaction between smoking and shared epitope genes in HLA-DR provides a high risk of seropositive rheumatoid arthritis. Arthritis and Rheumatism. 2004; **50**(10):3085-3092

[9] Klareskog L, Stolt P, Lundberg K, Källberg H, Bengtsson C, Grunewald J, et al. A new model for an etiology of rheumatoid arthritis: Smoking may trigger HLA-DR (shared epitope)-restricted immune reactions to autoantigens modified by citrullination. Arthritis and Rheumatism. 2006;**54**(1): 38-46

[10] Lundberg K, Wegner N, Yucel-Lindberg T, Venables PJ. Periodontitis in RA—The citrullinated enolase connection. Nature Reviews Rheumatology. 2010;**6**(12):727-730. DOI: 10.1038/nrrheum.2010.139

[11] Wegner N, Lundberg K, Kinloch A, Fisher B, Malmström V, Feldmann M, et al. Autoimmunity to specific citrullinated proteins gives the first clues to the etiology of rheumatoid arthritis. Immunological Reviews. 2010; **233**(1):34-54. DOI: 10.1111/j.0105 2896.2009.00850.x

[12] Shah HN, Collins MD. Proposal for reclassification of *Bacteroides asaccharolyticus*, *Bacteroides gingivalis*, and *Bacteroides endodontalis* in a new genus *Porphyromonas*. International

Journal of Systematic Bacteriology. 1988;**38**:128-131

[13] Lamont RJ, Koo H, Hajishengallis G. The Oral microbiota: Dynamic communities and host interactions. Nature Reviews. Microbiology. 2018 Dec;**16**(12):745-759. DOI: 10.1038/s41579-018-0089-x

[14] Konig MF, Abusleme L, Reinholdt J, Palmer RJ, Teles RP, Sampson K, et al. Aggregatibacter actinomy cetemcomitans-induced hypercitrullination links periodontal infection to autoimmunity in rheumatoid arthritis. Science Translational Medicine. 2016;**8**(369):369ra176. DOI: 10.1126/scitranslmed.aaj1921

[15] Snyderman R, McCarty GA. Analogous mechanisms of tissue destruction in rheumatoid arthritis and periodontal disease. In: Genco RJ, Mergenhagen SE, editors. Host-Parasite Interactions in Periodontal Diseases. Washington, DC, USA: American Society of Microbiology; 1982. pp. 354-362

[16] McGraw WT, Potempa J, Farley D, Travis J. Purification, characterization, and sequence analysis of a potential virulence factor from *Porphyromonas gingivalis*, peptidylarginine deiminase. Infection and Immunity. 1999;**67**(7):3248-3256

[17] Rosenstein ED, Greenwald RA, Kushner LJ, Weissmann G. Hypothesis: The humoral immune response to oral bacteria provides a stimulus for the development of rheumatoid arthritis. Inflammation. 2004;**28**(6):311-318. DOI: 10.1007/s10753-004-6641-z

[18] de Smit MJ, Brouwer E, Vissink A, van Winkelhoff AJ. Rheumatoid arthritis and periodontitis; a possible link via citrullination. Anaerobe. 2011;**17**(4):196-200. DOI: 10.1016/j.anaerobe.2011.03.019 Epub 2011 Apr 16

[19] Gómez-Bañuelos E, Mukherjee A, Darrah E, Andrade F. Rheumatoid arthritis-associated mechanisms of *Porphyromonas gingivalis* and *Aggregatibacter actinomycetemcomitans*. Journal of Clinical Medicine. 2019;**8**(9):1309. DOI: 10.3390/jcm8091309

[20] Feldmann M, Maini SR. Role of cytokines in rheumatoid arthritis: An education in pathophysiology and therapeutics. Immunological Reviews. 2008;**223**:7-19. DOI: 10.1111/j.1600-065X.2008.00626.x

[21] Fries JF. Current treatment paradigms in rheumatoid arthritis. Rheumatology (Oxford, England). 2000;**39**(Suppl 1):30-35

[22] Takayanagi H. Osteoimmunology and the effects of the immune system on bone. Nature Reviews Rheumatology. 2009;**5**(12):667-676. DOI: 10.1038/nrrheum.2009.217

[23] Lucchino B, Spinelli FR, Iannuccelli C, Guzzo MP, Conti F, Di Franco M. Mucosa-environment interactions in the pathogenesis of rheumatoid arthritis. Cell. 2019;**8**(7):700. DOI: 10.3390/cells8070700

[24] Catrina AI, Svensson CI, Malmström V, Schett G, Klareskog L. Mechanisms leading from systemic autoimmunity to joint-specific disease in rheumatoid arthritis. Nature Reviews Rheumatology. 2017;**13**(2):79-86. DOI: 10.1038/nrrheum.2016.200

[25] Visser K, van der Heijde D. Optimal dosage and route of administration of methotrexate in rheumatoid arthritis: A systematic review of the literature. Annals of the Rheumatic Diseases. 2009;**68**(7):1094-1099. DOI: 10.1136/ard.2008.092668

[26] Wasserman AM. Diagnosis and management of rheumatoid arthritis.

American Family Physician. 2011; **84**(11):1245-1252

[27] Smolen JS, Aletaha D. Rheumatoid arthritis therapy reappraisal: Strategies, opportunities and challenges. Nature Reviews Rheumatology. 2015;**11**(5): 276-289. DOI: 10.1038/nrrheum.2015.8

[28] Ramiro S, Gaujoux-Viala C, Nam JL, Smolen JS, Buch M, Gossec L, et al. Safety of synthetic and biological DMARDs: A systematic literature review informing the 2013 update of the EULAR recommendations for management of rheumatoid arthritis. Annals of the Rheumatic Diseases. 2014; **73**(3):529-535. DOI: 10.1136/ annrheumdis-2013-204575

[29] Smolen JS, Landewé R, Breedveld FC, Dougados M, Emery P, Gaujoux-Viala C, et al. EULAR recommendations for the management of rheumatoid arthritis with synthetic and biological disease-modifying antirheumatic drugs. Annals of the Rheumatic Diseases. 2010;**69**(6): 964-975. DOI: 10.1136/ard.2009.126532. Review. Erratum in: Ann Rheum Dis. 2011 Aug;70(8):1519

[30] Smolen JS, Landewé R, Breedveld FC, Buch M, Burmester G, Dougados M, et al. EULAR recommendations for the management of rheumatoid arthritis with synthetic and biological disease-modifying antirheumatic drugs: 2013 update. Annals of the Rheumatic Diseases. 2014; **73**(3):492-509. DOI: 10.1136/ annrheumdis-2013-204573

[31] Smolen JS, Landewé R, Bijlsma J, Burmester G, Chatzidionysiou K, Dougados M, et al. EULAR recommendations for the management of rheumatoid arthritis with synthetic and biological disease-modifying antirheumatic drugs: 2016 update. Annals of the Rheumatic Diseases. 2017; **76**(6):960-977. DOI: 10.1136/ annrheumdis-2016-210715

[32] Smolen JS, Landewé RBM, Bijlsma JWJ, Burmester GR, Dougados M, Kerschbaumer A, et al. EULAR recommendations for the management of rheumatoid arthritis with synthetic and biological disease-modifying antirheumatic drugs: 2019 update. Annals of the Rheumatic Diseases. 2020. DOI: 10.1136/ annrheumdis-2019-216655

[33] Baker JF, Ostergaard M, Emery P, Hsia EC, Lu J, Baker DG, et al. Early MRI measures independently predict 1-year and 2-year radiographic progression in rheumatoid arthritis: Secondary analysis from a large clinical trial. Annals of the Rheumatic Diseases. 2014;**73**(11):1968-1974. DOI: 10.1136/ annrheumdis-2013-203444

[34] Smolen JS, Aletaha D, Barton A, Burmester GR, Emery P, Firestein GS, et al. Rheumatoid arthritis. Nature Reviews. Disease Primers. 2018;**4**: 18001. DOI: 10.1038/nrdp.2018.1

[35] Migita K, Izumi Y, Torigoshi T, Satomura K, Izumi M, Nishino Y, et al. Inhibition of Janus kinase/signal transducer and activator of transcription (JAK/STAT) signalling pathway in rheumatoid synovial fibroblasts using small molecule compounds. Clinical and Experimental Immunology. 2013;**174**(3):356-363. DOI: 10.1111/cei.12190

[36] O'Shea JJ, Schwartz DM, Villarino AV, Gadina M, McInnes IB, Laurence A. The JAK-STAT pathway: Impact on human disease and therapeutic intervention. Annual Review of Medicine. 2015;**66**:311-328. DOI: 10.1146/annurev-med-051113-024537

[37] Taylor PC. Clinical efficacy of launched JAK inhibitors in rheumatoid arthritis. Rheumatology (Oxford, England). 2019;**58**(Suppl 1):i17-i26. DOI: 10.1093/rheumatology/key225

[38] Smolen JS, Landewé RBM, Bijlsma JWJ, Burmester GR, Dougados M, Kerschbaumer A, et al. EULAR recommendations for the management of rheumatoid arthritis with synthetic and biological disease-modifying antirheumatic drugs: 2019 update. Annals of the Rheumatic Diseases. 2020. DOI: 10.1136/annrheumdis-2019-216655

[39] van der Woude D, van der Helm-van Mil AHM. Update on the epidemiology, risk factors, and disease outcomes of rheumatoid arthritis. Best Practice & Research. Clinical Rheumatology. 2018;**32**(2):174-187. DOI: 10.1016/j.berh.2018.10.005

[40] Sugimoto H, Takeda A, Masuyama J, Furuse M. Early-stage rheumatoid arthritis: Diagnostic accuracy of MR imaging. Radiology. 1996;**198**(1):185-192

[41] Sugimoto H, Takeda A, Kano S. Assessment of disease activity in rheumatoid arthritis using magnetic resonance imaging: Quantification of pannus volume in the hands. British Journal of Rheumatology. 1998;**37**(8):854-861

[42] Sugimoto H, Takeda A, Hyodoh K. Early-stage rheumatoid arthritis: Prospective study of the effectiveness of MR imaging for diagnosis. Radiology. 2000;**216**(2):569-575

[43] Sugimoto H, Takeda A, Hyodoh K. MR imaging for evaluation of early rheumatoid arthritis. Seminars in Musculoskeletal Radiology. June 2001;5 (2):159-165

[44] Aggarwal R, Ringold S, Khanna D, Neogi T, Johnson SR, Miller A, et al. Distinctions between diagnostic and classification criteria? Arthritis Care & Research. 2015;**67**(7):891-897. DOI: 10.1002/acr.22583

[45] Arnett FC, Edworthy SM, Bloch DA, McShane DJ, Fries JF, Cooper NS, et al. The American Rheumatism Association 1987 revised criteria for the classification of rheumatoid arthritis. Arthritis and Rheumatism. 1988;**31**(3):315-324

[46] Banal F, Dougados M, Combescure C, Gossec L. Sensitivity and specificity of the American College of Rheumatology 1987 criteria for the diagnosis of rheumatoid arthritis according to disease duration: A systematic literature review and meta-analysis. Annals of the Rheumatic Diseases. 2009;**68**(7):1184-1191. DOI: 10.1136/ard.2008.093187

[47] Harrison BJ, Symmons DP, Barrett EM, Silman AJ. The performance of the 1987 ARA classification criteria for rheumatoid arthritis in a population based cohort of patients with early inflammatory polyarthritis. American Rheumatism Association. Journal of Rheumatology. 1998;**25**(12):2324-2330

[48] Aletaha D, Neogi T, Silman AJ, Funovits J, Felson DT, Bingham CO 3rd, et al. 2010 rheumatoid arthritis classification criteria: An American College of Rheumatology/European League Against Rheumatism collaborative initiative. Annals of the Rheumatic Diseases. 2010;**69**(9): 1580-1588. DOI: 10.1136/ard.2010.138461

[49] Shmerling RH, Delbanco TL. The rheumatoid factor: An analysis of clinical utility. The American Journal of Medicine. 1991;**91**(5):528-534

[50] Ingegnoli F, Castelli R, Gualtierotti R. Rheumatoid factors: Clinical applications. Disease Markers. 2013;**35**(6):727-734. DOI: 10.1155/2013/726598

[51] Aggarwal R, Liao K, Nair R, Ringold S, Costenbader KH. Anti-citrullinated peptide antibody assays and their role in the diagnosis of

rheumatoid arthritis. Arthritis and Rheumatism. 2009;**61**(11):1472-1483. DOI: 10.1002/art.24827

[52] Scott DL, Wolfe F, Huizinga TW. Rheumatoid arthritis. Lancet. 2010; **376**(9746):1094-1108. DOI: 10.1016/S0140-6736(10)60826-4

[53] Kaneko Y, Kuwana M, Kameda H, Takeuchi T. Sensitivity and specificity of 2010 rheumatoid arthritis classification criteria. Rheumatology (Oxford, England). 2011;**50**(7): 1268-1274. DOI: 10.1093/rheumatology/keq442

[54] Aletaha D, Eberl G, Nell VP, Machold KP, Smolen JS. Practical progress in realisation of early diagnosis and treatment of patients with suspected rheumatoid arthritis: Results from two matched questionnaires within three years. Annals of the Rheumatic Diseases. 2002;**61**(7): 630-634

[55] Alarcón GS, Koopman WJ, Acton RT, Barger BO. Seronegative rheumatoid arthritis. A distinct immunogenetic disease? Arthritis and Rheumatism. 1982;**25**(5):502-507

[56] McGonagle D, Conaghan PG, Wakefield R, Emery P. Imaging the joints in early rheumatoid arthritis. Best Practice & Research. Clinical Rheumatology. 2001;**15**(1):91-104

[57] Schild HH. MRI Made Easy (...well almost). Berlin: Schering; 1990

[58] Østergaard M, Peterfy C, Conaghan P, McQueen F, Bird P, Ejbjerg B, et al. OMERACT Rheumatoid Arthritis magnetic resonance imaging studies. Core set of MRI acquisitions, joint pathology definitions, and the OMERACT RA-MRI scoring system. The Journal of Rheumatology. 2003; **30**(6):1385-1386

[59] Tamai K, Yamato M, Yamaguchi T, Ohno W. Dynamic magnetic resonance imaging for the evaluation of synovitis in patients with rheumatoid arthritis. Arthritis and Rheumatism. 1994;**37**(8): 1151-1157

[60] Yamato M, Tamai K, Yamaguchi T, Ohno W. MRI of the knee in rheumatoid arthritis: Gd-DTPA perfusion dynamics. Journal of Computer Assisted Tomography. 1993;**17**(5):781-785

[61] Nakahara N, Uetani M, Hayashi K, Kawahara Y, Matsumoto T, Oda J. Gadolinium-enhanced MR imaging of the wrist in rheumatoid arthritis: Value of fat suppression pulse sequences. Skeletal Radiology. 1996;**25**(7):639-647

[62] Schumacher HR. Primer on the Rheumatic Diseases. 10th ed. Atlanta: Arthritis Foundation; 1993. p. 99

Chapter 2

Lupus Erythematosus: Dermatologic Perspectives on the Diversity

Ran Xin, Wang Peng, Huang Jinghong, Pradhan Sushmita, Yang Heli and Ran Yuping

Abstract

Lupus is one of the complex autoimmune disease, which is difficult to diagnose and consists of few subtypes that are required to be classified. During our clinical work, we found out that the dermoscopy can be of great benefit to diagnose discoid lupus erythematosus (DLE). The histopathological examination is very important to confirm the diagnosis. The cases of infant LE patients, may derive the autoimmune antibodies from their mothers in order to diagnose the neonatal lupus erythematosus. Thus, it is very important to examine the antibodies of the mother, who may also be a subclinical LE patient and need continuous follow-ups or even treatment managements. Here, we present the cases of lupus with particular characteristics including linear cutaneous lupus erythematosus, DLE, and neonatal lupus erythematosus.

Keywords: lupus erythematosus, linear erythematous atrophic patch, neonatal lupus erythematosus, discoid lupus erythematosus, dermoscopy

1. Introduction

Systemic lupus erythematosus is a chronic, relapsing, inflammatory, and often febrile multisystemic disorder of the connective tissue, characterized principally by involvement of the skin, joints, kidneys, and serosal membranes. The word lupus means wolf in Latin, as the destructive injuries the disease caused brought to mind the bites of this animal [1, 2]. The earliest usage of the term lupus in the English literature is in the tenth century biography of St. Martin, written in 963 AD. However, the modern period of our understanding of this disease began in 1948, when Mayo Clinic hematologist Malcolm Hargraves [3] discovered the LE cell.

Lupus is all known as a spectrum disease, the symptoms between patients varies from mild to severe and can be divided into systemic lupus erythematosus (SLE) and cutaneous lupus erythematosus (CLE). CLE includes three subsets of LE-specific skin diseases: acute cutaneous lupus erythematosus (ACLE), subacute cutaneous lupus erythematosus (SCLE), and chronic cutaneous lupus erythematosus (CCLE). CCLE encompasses discoid lupus erythematosus (DLE), lupus erythematosus tumidus (LE tumidus), lupus profundus (also known as lupus panniculitis), chilblain lupus erythematosus (chilblain LE), and lichenoid cutaneous lupus erythematosus-lichen planus overlap syndrome

(LE-LP overlap syndrome). CLE can occur as a manifestation of SLE or independent of SLE. Patients with SLE may also develop a variety of LE-nonspecific skin diseases, cutaneous disorders that lack histologic features of LE, but occur with increased frequency in patients with SLE.

On diagnosing a systemic lupus erythematosus, we have several groups of diagnostic criteria. The major positive characteristics such as swollen joints, butterfly rash on the face, photo-sensitivity, or hair loss helps in the confirmation of the diagnosis. The laboratory examinations such as double-stranded DNA antibody (ds-DNA), anti-nuclear antibody (ANA) and other autoimmune antibodies are regarded as the highest level of consideration.

A systematic approach should be taken because of the diversity and complexity of clinical and laboratory manifestations [4–6]. Clinical manifestations may be due to one or any combination of the following: disease activity from active inflammation or thrombosis, acute drug toxicity, chronic damage due to the effects of the disease or its treatment (such as lung fibrosis or atherosclerosis), or comorbidity (e.g., infection). It is important to take a detailed history and to perform a clinical examination, including vital signs and urinalysis, to establish the likely differential diagnoses and then to organize the relevant investigations, depending on the circumstances. In addition, when assessing disease activity with a view to planning treatment, it is necessary to determine the circumstances that may have led to a lupus flare (such as exposure to sunlight, infection, hormonal changes, or previous disease-related therapeutic change) as this will guide further investigation, treatment change and disease monitoring required thereafter.

However, there are many subtypes of lupus, such as discoid lupus erythematosus and neonatal lupus erythematosus that does not follow the standard diagnostic criterion. Here, we present four instructive case studies of lupus. We hope this chapter will enlighten the perspective on lupus.

2. Brief overview of dermoscopy

Dermoscopy is a noninvasive method that allows the *in vivo* evaluation of colors and microstructures of the epidermis. It has been widely studied in differentiating benign and malignant skin lesions. With dermoscopy the diagnostician's sensitivity to diagnose melanoma is 90% compared to 74% when the technique is not used. It helps to avoid unnecessary surgery and give dermatologist more perspectives to plan the surgery. The diagnose and differential diagnosis of hair and nail diseases are also getting advanced benefits since application of dermoscopy. And now, dermoscopy is expanding its role as a tool for the evaluation of inflammatory skin conditions such as psoriasis, lichen planus and lupus.

3. Case presentations

3.1 Case 1. Linear cutaneous lupus erythematosus distributed along a reverse Blaschko lines

A 15-year-old female presented with itching linear erythema on the left forehead for 3 years. The erythema extended gradually to the scalp and the left upper eyelid, distributed in a linear pattern over time [7]. The patient was healthy except the lesion. Family history was negative. Physical examination showed that she was in good conditions. Dermatological examinations showed a longitudinal erythema on the left side of the hairline, forehead and left upper eyelid distributed in "S" shape pattern. The surface of forehead lesion showed obvious atrophy, telangiectasis and adhesive scales (**Figure 1a**).

Laboratory examination of routine blood and urine test results, liver and renal function were all normal. Serum IgG, IgA, IgM, IgE, rheumatoid factor (RF), CIC, ANA, Anti-ds-DNA, Anti-RNP, Anti-SM, SSA, SSB, Anti-SCL-70 and Anti-Jo-1 antibody were within normal limits. Complement 3 (C_3) 0.749 g/L (normal value, 0.785–1.52 g/L), Complement 4 (C_4) 0.121 g/L (normal value, 0.145–0.36 g/L). Histological examination showed follicular keratotic plugging, vacuolar alteration of the basal cell layer, thickening of the basement membrane, perivascular infiltration of lymphocytes in the dermis (**Figure 1b** and **c**), which led to the diagnosis of linear cutaneous lupus erythematosus.

She was treated with compound glycyrrhizin tablets (two tablets three times a day, containing 150 mg glycyrrhizin, 210 mg monoammonium glycyrrhizinate, 150 mg aminoacetic acid, and 150 mg methionine), hydroxychloroquine tablets (200 mg once a day), and topical application of 0.1% tacrolimus ointment (twice a day). After half a year of follow-up, the skin lesion was improved with no tendency of systemic involvement.

3.2 Case 2. Dermoscopic presentation of DLE

A 38-year-old male with rapidly progressing papules demonstrating the features of acne on the left prefrontal region accompanied with tenderness for 2 months (**Figure 2a**). The patient had been diagnosed as epifolliculitis and treated with mupirocin cream for 1 month with no improvement. Physical examination revealed erythema, papules, callus shells, and plaques on his left prefrontal region. The results of blood routine and serum immunological examinations were normal. The specificity examinations including circulating immune complex, C_3 and C_4, antinuclear antibodies, double-stranded DNA antibody (ds-DNA), SSA/Ro antibody, and SSB/La antibody showed no any significant findings. However, dermoscopy of the lesions showed that the erythematous base was interrupted by a prominent keratinization around the hair follicles and follicular keratotic plugging (**Figure 2b**) [8]. It clued for differentiating atypical discoid lupus erythematosus from epifolliculitis with dermoscopy, and dermoscopy guided biopsy yielded a definitive histopathological diagnosis of the case. Histopathological evaluation of the lesions revealed dilated follicular openings filled with cornified material, follicular plugging, a necrosed part of the stratum basale, and inflammatory cell infiltration of the perifollicular and shallow dermal layers, which indicated discoid

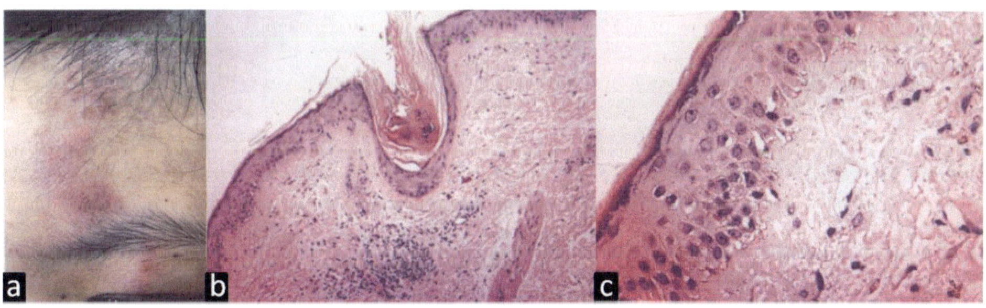

Figure 1.
(a) A longitudinal erythema on the left side of the hairline, forehead and left upper eyelid distributed in an "S" pattern. The forehead lesion showed obvious atrophy, telangiectasis and adhesive scales. (b) Histological examination showed epidermal atrophy, follicular plugging, and the perivascular infiltration of lymphocytes in the dermis (HE stain × 100). (c) Vacuolar alteration in the basal layer of the epidermis, and thickening of the basement membrane (HE stain × 400).

lupus erythematosus (**Figure 2c**). The diagnosis of discoid lupus erythematosus (DLE) was confirmed. The patient received hydroxychloroquine 200 mg once a day, compound glycyrrhizin tablets (two tablets three times a day, containing 150 mg glycyrrhizin, 210 mg monoammonium glycyrrhizinate, 150 mg amino-acetic acid, and 150 mg methionine), and topical application of 0.1% tacrolimus cream once a day. The condition of the patient improved after 4 months of treatment (**Figure 2d** and **e**).

3.3 Case 3. Neonatal lupus erythematosus

A 3-month-old female infant presented with a butterfly-like edematous erythematosus on the center of her face, with raised border and scales (**Figure 3a**).

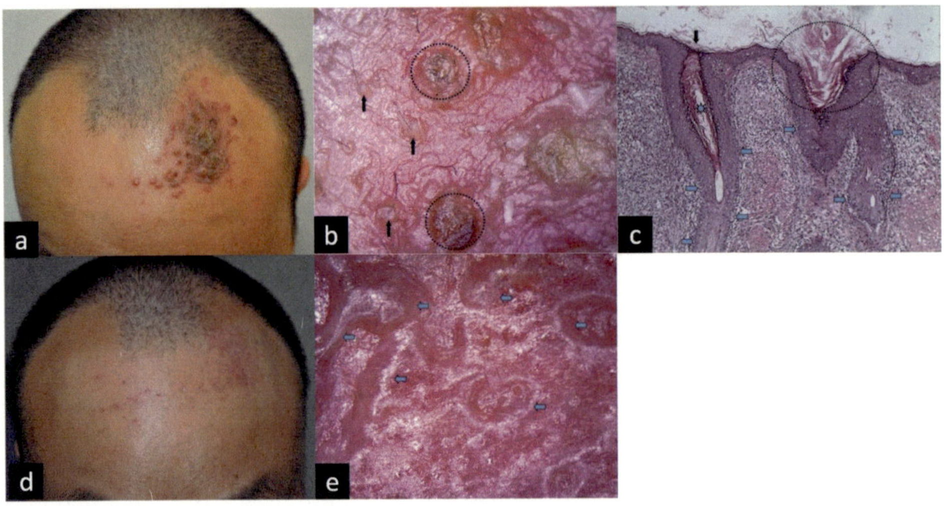

Figure 2.
(a) A 38-year-old male showed erythema, papules, callus shells, and plaques on the left prefrontal region. (b) Dermoscopic evaluation of the lesions showed an erythematosus base interrupted by keratinization around the hair follicles and follicular keratotic plugging. (c) Histopathologic evaluation of the lesions revealed dilated follicular openings filled with cornified material, follicular plugging, a necrosed part of the stratum basale, and inflammatory cell infiltration of the perifollicular and shallow dermal layers, which indicated discoid lupus erythematosus (DLE) (HE stain, original magnification × 40). (d) After more than 4 months of treatment, the condition improved obviously. (e) Dermoscopic evaluation of the lesions showed an erythematosus scar instead of keratinization around the hair follicles, and follicular keratotic plugging.

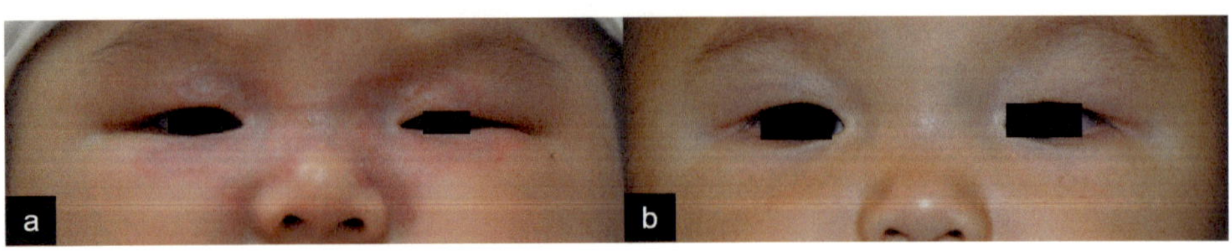

Figure 3.
(a) A 3-month-old female infant presented with butterfly-like edematous erythematosus on the center of her face, with raised border and scales. (b) After continuous treatment for 153 days with 0.03% tacrolimus cream once a day, and total glucosides of paeony capsules 300 mg once a day, the butterfly-like rash almost disappeared.

Due to the presence of scales on the lesion, a direct microscope examination with 16% potassium hydroxide (KOH), was done to rule out the fungal infection. However, the examination was not significant. In order to rule out congenital syphilis, the *Treponema pallidum* particle agglutination assay (TPPA) and toluidine red unheated serum test (TRUST) tests were also done, with negative results. Finally, the autoimmune antibodies were examined. The report showed ANA (±), Anti-SSA (+++), and C_3 and C_4 were reduced. However, Anti-ds-DNA and rest of the anti-ENA examinations were not significant. The autoimmune antibodies of the patient's mother were not significant. The report showed ANA (+), Anti-SSA (+++) and Anti-Ro-52 (+++). Based on the manifestations, the final diagnosis of neonatal lupus erythematosus (NLE) was confirmed. The patient was treated with topical application of 0.03% tacrolimus cream once a day and total glucosides of paeony capsules 300 mg once a day.

After continuous treatment for 153 days, the butterfly-like rash almost disappeared (**Figure 3b**). After following up for 5 years, the conditions of both the patient and her mother improved with no features of lupus erythematosus.

3.4 Case 4. Neonatal lupus erythematosus baby and her SCLE mother

A 3-month-old female infant presented with butterfly-like rash on the center of her face since birth (**Figure 4a**). The dermoscopy of the lesion showed perifollicular whitish halo and telangiectasias (**Figure 4b**). It was quite similar with the most common dermoscopic criteria of LE.

Meanwhile while examining the mother's face, we found pink-red erythematous plaque on the center of her face (**Figure 4c**), which may get worse after sun exposure. And also, we found red edematous coin shaped patch on the left side of her face. Dermoscopy of the skin lesion showed typical telangiectasias manifestations (**Figure 4d**).

The autoimmune antibodies examinations of the infant showed ANA (1:100), Anti-SSA (+), C_3 and C_4 were reduced. And her mother's examination showed ANA (1:1000), Anti-SSA (+++), C_3 and C_4 were reduced. However, the ds-DNA and the rest of anti-ENA examinations were not significant.

The final diagnosis of the infant as neonatal lupus erythematosus (NLE), and her mother as SCLE were confirmed.

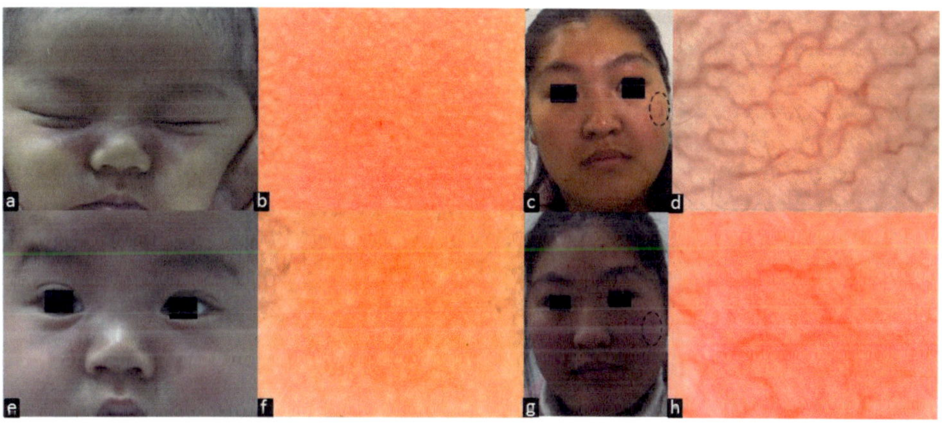

Figure 4.
(a) A 3-month-old female infant presented with butterfly-like rash on the center of her face since birth. (b) Dermoscopy showed perifollicular whitish halo and telangiectasias with a pink-red background. (c) The mother's face showed pink-red erythematous plaques on the center of her face, which may get worse after sun exposure. (d) Dermoscopy of the skin lesion showed typical telangiectasias manifestations with a pink-red background. (e) After 125 days follow up without medication, the baby's butterfly-like rash almost disappeared. (f) Dermoscopy showed the red background of lesion was lighter than initial performance. (g) After treatment for 125 days with 30 mg prednisone once a day, the skin lesion of the mother subsided. (h) Dermoscopy showed improved manifestations of telangiectasias.

The infant was given total paeony glycoside orally, but her parents did not implement it to her actually. The mother was treated with 30 mg prednisone once a day and was recommended to protect the skin from excessive sun exposure. The butterfly like rash of the baby almost disappeared when the follow-up after 125 days (**Figure 4e** and **f**), and the results of immunological examination were within the normal range. The skin lesion of the mother subsided (**Figure 4g** and **h**) and the re-examination of her autoimmune antibodies' examinations showed ANA (1:1000), Anti-SSA (+++) with no symptoms.

4. Discussion

Linear cutaneous lupus erythematosus (LCLE) is rare, and the skin lesions are mostly distributed along the Blaschko lines. The Blaschko lines, which was first described by and named by Blaschko in 1901, is the special lines on the surface of the human body. On the back of the trunk, the Blaschko line is V-shaped across the spine, and S-shaped on the anterior and lateral skins of the trunk. It exists in the form of vertical stripes on the skin of extremities, and is turbine-like on the surface of the abdominal skin and spiral-like on the scalp. The schematic diagram of the division of the facial Blaschko line was proposed see [9] in 1994, and it has different distribution patterns in different parts of the face. Discoid lupus erythematosus (DLE) lesion distribute along the Blaschko line in two Japanese children with the onset age being 3 and 11 years and the lesions located in the right cheek, left lower jaw and left neck, respectively in 1998 [10]. The authors analyzed the previous 6 cases and the current 2 cases, whereby they found that the 6 patients had an onset age of being smaller than 14 years, and that none of the patients had progressed into systemic lupus erythematosus. They argued that it might be a new subtype of lupus erythematosus, and proposed the name of linear cutaneous lupus erythematosus for DLE lesion with a linear configuration. In 1999 subsequently, an 8-year-old black boy with a lesion of LCLE along the Blaschko line in the right cheek and right chest, respectively see [11]; a 3-year-old Hispanic boy developed a lesion on his face and neck in 2002 see [12]. The lesion in our patient was located in the left forehead and left upper eyelid, which was formed S-shaped lesion, but was not distributed along the Blaschko line. This case was rather rarer and indicated that the skin lesion of LCLE was not necessarily distributed along the Blaschko line. In an adult case with linear, atrophic, plaque on left jaw and neck which did not follow the lines of Blaschko strictly [13]. But our case followed a reversed Blaschko lines (S shape line) on the left face.

As a matter of fact, the clinical presentations of DLE could be difficult to distinguish from other erythematous like patches and plaques. Thus, we highly recommend the use of non-invasive tool of dermoscopic technology to examine the details of skin lesions. The manifestations under dermoscopic findings of DLE could have erythematous base interrupted by prominent keratinization around the hair follicles and follicular keratotic plugging. According to the studies, follicular keratotic plug is one of the markers of discoid lupus erythematosus [14].

Another important method to confirm the diagnosis of DLE is histopathological examination. The typical features of DLE is follicular keratotic plugging, vacuolar alteration of the basal cell layer, thickening of the basement membrane, perivascular and periappendicular infiltration of the lymphocytes in the dermis.

Autoimmune antibodies such as Anti-Ds-DNA, ANA, ENA and immunoglobulins plays an important role in the diagnosis of SLE patients. However, in most conditions, the positive rate of antibodies could be very low in DLE patients. And in some patients no any manifestations are seen except the skin lesions.

SLE in children is fundamentally the same disease as in adults, with similar etiology, pathogenesis, clinical manifestations, and laboratory findings. However, it is generally accepted that children with SLE have greater disease severity and earlier accrual of disease damage than adults with SLE [15–19]. Worldwide, estimates of childhood-onset SLE incidence are between 0.3 and 2.2 per 100,000 children-years, while prevalence rates range widely from 3.3 to 9.7 per 100,000 children and adolescents, depending upon the population studied and its ethnic distribution [20–31].

Neonatal lupus is a rare syndrome that is associated with maternal antibodies to Ro/SSA, to La/SSB, and, much less frequently, to U1RNP. Infants develop eruptions characterized by erythematous arcuate patches or plaques with raised active margins shortly after birth. Congenital heart block is the most concerning complication of neonatal lupus. Following the birth of an infant with neonatal lupus, the risk for congenital heart block is increased with subsequent pregnancies [32]. Of note, treatment with hydroxychloroquine may decrease the risk of neonatal lupus (congenital heart block) in at-risk pregnancies [33].

The infant LE patients may derive the autoimmune antibodies from their mother in order to diagnose the neonatal lupus erythematosus. Thus, it is very important to examine the antibodies of the mother, who may also be a subclinical LE patient and need continuous follow-ups or managements.

For treatment, topical application of tacrolimus ointment is the most recommended therapy. Except one SCLE patient who had significantly increase titers of ANA and Anti-SSA, we used mild moderate dose of prednisone, all other LCLE, DLE and NLE did not give systemic prednisone, instead with compound glycyrrhizin tablets, or, total glucosides of paeony capsules which made from the extracts of traditional Chinese medicine. During our clinical practices, these medicines showed reliable efficiency and very few of side effect, with a favorable prognosis. In case 4, the skin lesion of neonatal lupus erythematosus baby spontaneously alleviated, suggested that it can remission without disposal, accompanied the autoantibodies from her mother decreases. But long-term follow-up is still needed.

5. Conclusion

In order to confirm the special clinical cases of lupus, such as linear cutaneous lupus erythematosus, DLE, or neonatal lupus erythematosus, the characteristics of dermoscopy and autoimmune antibodies tests are important. In these cases, topical tacrolimus, oral compound glycyrrhizin or total paeony glycoside, or, hydroxychloroquine had good prognosis, without systemic glucocorticoid therapy.

Acknowledgements

No funding.

Conflict of interest

No conflict of interest.

Author details

Ran Xin, Wang Peng, Huang Jinghong, Pradhan Sushmita, Yang Heli and Ran Yuping*
Department of Dermatovenereology, West China Hospital, Sichuan University, Chengdu, China

*Address all correspondence to: ranyuping@vip.sina.com

References

[1] Blotzer JW. Systemic lupus erythematosus I: Historical aspects. Maryland State Medical Journal. 1983;**32**:439-441

[2] Holubar K. Terminology and iconography of lupus erythematosus: A historical vignette. The American Journal of Dermatopathology. 1980;**2**:239-242

[3] Hargraves MM. Discovery of the LE cell and its morphology. Mayo Clinic Proceedings. 1969;**44**:579-599

[4] Kumar K, Chambers S, Gordon C. Challenges of ethnicity in SLE. Best Practice and Research. Clinical Rheumatology. 2009;**23**:549-561

[5] The American College of Rheumatology nomenclature and case definitions for neuropsychiatric lupus syndromes. Arthritis and Rheumatism. 1999;**42**:599-608

[6] Bertsias GK, Boumpas DT. Pathogenesis, diagnosis and management of neuropsychiatric SLE manifestations. Nature Reviews Rheumatology. 2010;**6**:358-367

[7] Wang P, Ran YP. Linear discoid lupus erythematosus: A case report. Journal of Clinical Dermatology. 2011;**40**(12):742-743 (In Chinese)

[8] Huang JH, Tang JQ, Ran YP. Indicators for differentiating atypical discoid lupus erythematosus from epifolliculitis with dermoscopy. Chinese Medical Journal. 2016;**129**(10):1255-1256. DOI: 10.4103/0366-6999.181953

[9] Bolognia JL, Orlow SJ, Glick SA. Lines of Blaschko. Journal of the American Academy of Dermatology. 1994;**31**(2 Pt 1):157-190

[10] Abe M, Ishikawa O, Miyachi Y. Linear cutaneous lupus erythematosus following the lines of Blaschko. The British Journal of Dermatology. 1998;**139**(2):307-310

[11] Green JJ, Baker DJ. Linear childhood discoid lupus erythematosus following the lines of Blaschko: A case report with review of the linear manifestations of lupus erythematosus. Pediatric Dermatology. 1999;**16**(2):128-133

[12] Requena C, Torrelo A, de Prada I, et al. Linear childhood cutaneous lupus erythematosus following Blaschko lines. Journal of the European Academy of Dermatology and Venereology. 2002;**16**(6):618-620

[13] Mao QX, Zhang WL, Wang Q, et al. Linear cutaneous lupus erythematosus/discoid lupus erythematosus in an adult. Postępy Dermatologii i Alergologii. 2017;**34**(2):177-179. DOI: 10.5114/ada.2017.67086. Epub: 13 April 2017

[14] Lopez-Tinos BO, Garcia-Hidalgo L, Orozco-Topete R. Dermoscopy in active discoid lupus. Archives of Dermatology. 2009;**145**:358. DOI: 10.1001/archdermatol.2008.585

[15] das Chagas Medeiros MM, Bezerra MC, Braga FN, et al. Clinical and immunological aspects and outcome of a Brazilian cohort of 414 patients with systemic lupus erythematosus (SLE): Comparison between childhood-onset, adult-onset, and late-onset SLE. Lupus. 2016;**25**:355

[16] Tucker LB, Menon S, Schaller JG, Isenberg DA. Adult- and childhood-onset systemic lupus erythematosus: A comparison of onset, clinical features, serology, and outcome. British Journal of Rheumatology. 1995;**34**:866

[17] Brunner HI, Gladman DD, Ibañez D, et al. Difference in disease features between childhood-onset and adult-onset systemic lupus erythematosus. Arthritis and Rheumatism. 2008;**58**:556

[18] Hersh AO, von Scheven E, Yazdany J, et al. Differences in long-term disease activity and treatment of adult patients with childhood- and adult-onset systemic lupus erythematosus. Arthritis and Rheumatism. 2009;**61**:13

[19] Hoffman IE, Lauwerys BR, De Keyser F, et al. Juvenile-onset systemic lupus erythematosus: Different clinical and serological pattern than adult-onset systemic lupus erythematosus. Annals of the Rheumatic Diseases. 2009;**68**:412

[20] Mackie FE, Kainer G, Adib N, et al. The national incidence and clinical picture of SLE in children in Australia—A report from the Australian paediatric surveillance unit. Lupus. 2015;**24**:66

[21] Huang JL, Yao TC, See LC. Prevalence of pediatric systemic lupus erythematosus and juvenile chronic arthritis in a Chinese population: A nation-wide prospective population-based study in Taiwan. Clinical and Experimental Rheumatology. 2004;**22**:776

[22] Al-Arfaj AS, Al-Balla SR, Al-Dalaan AN, et al. Prevalence of systemic lupus erythematosus in central Saudi Arabia. Saudi Medical Journal. 2002;**23**:87

[23] Hiraki LT, Feldman CH, Liu J, et al. Prevalence, incidence, and demographics of systemic lupus erythematosus and lupus nephritis from 2000 to 2004 among children in the US Medicaid beneficiary population. Arthritis and Rheumatism. 2012;**64**:2669

[24] Kamphuis S, Silverman ED. Prevalence and burden of pediatric-onset systemic lupus erythematosus. Nature Reviews Rheumatology. 2010;**6**:538

[25] Malleson PN, Fung MY, Rosenberg AM. The incidence of pediatric rheumatic diseases: Results from the Canadian Pediatric Rheumatology Association Disease Registry. The Journal of Rheumatology. 1996;**23**:1981

[26] Huemer C, Huemer M, Dorner T, et al. Incidence of pediatric rheumatic diseases in a regional population in Austria. The Journal of Rheumatology. 2001;**28**:2116

[27] Kurahara DK, Grandinetti A, Fujii LL, et al. Visiting consultant clinics to study prevalence rates of juvenile rheumatoid arthritis and childhood systemic lupus erythematosus across dispersed geographic areas. The Journal of Rheumatology. 2007;**34**:425

[28] Houghton KM, Page J, Cabral DA, et al. Systemic lupus erythematosus in the pediatric North American Native population of British Columbia. The Journal of Rheumatology. 2006;**33**:161

[29] Huang JL, Yeh KW, Yao TC, et al. Pediatric lupus in Asia. Lupus. 2010;**19**:1414

[30] Malaviya AN, Singh RR, Singh YN, et al. Prevalence of systemic lupus erythematosus in India. Lupus. 1993;**2**:115

[31] Chopra A. Disease burden of rheumatic diseases in India: COPCORD perspective. Indian Journal of Rheumatology. 2015;**10**:70

[32] Izmirly PM, Llanos C, Lee LA, et al. Cutaneous manifestations of neonatal lupus and risk of subsequent congenital heart block. Arthritis and Rheumatism. 2010;**62**:1153

[33] Izmirly PM, Costedoat-Chalumeau N, Pisoni CN, et al. Maternal use of hydroxychloroquine is associated with a reduced risk of recurrent anti-SSA/Ro-antibody-associated cardiac manifestations of neonatal lupus. Circulation. 2012;**126**:76

Chapter 3

The Established and Evolving Role of Nailfold Capillaroscopy in Connective-Tissue Disease

Matthew J.S. Parker and Neil W. McGill

Abstract

Nailfold capillaroscopy (NFC) is a low-cost, non-invasive, rapid, highly specific and reproducible investigation well established in the diagnosis of systemic sclerosis and related conditions. This chapter will detail the relevant underlying scientific principles that underpin the investigation, the methods for performing NFC, the range of abnormalities that can be present and the currently available classification criteria before moving on to discuss the various established and emerging applications as relevant to the connective tissue diseases. In addition to its role in the diagnosis of SSc, highlighted by its inclusion in the most recent ACR/EULAR consensus classification criteria, NFC has been shown to predict disease activity, many organ-specific complications such as digital ulcers, pulmonary hypertension and interstitial lung disease, and even mortality. It is emerging as a useful investigation in other CTDs characterised by microvasculopathy, such as in the idiopathic inflammatory myopathies and mixed connective tissue disease, as well as being studied as a serial investigation in patients to act as a potential biomarker and measure of treatment efficacy. NFC can contribute to the earlier identification of patients with CTDs with clinically important complications and if applied accurately, therefore, can help improve outcomes in these often challenging diseases.

Keywords: nailfold capillaroscopy, systemic sclerosis, polymyositis, dermatomyositis

1. Introduction

The technique of nailfold capillaroscopy (NFC) was first described almost 100 years ago by Brown and O'Leary, but its utility in connective tissue disease was first truly recognised and demonstrated through the work of Maricq et al. in the 1970s and 1980s [1–3]. It is now established as a low-cost, non-invasive, highly specific, reproducible, and rapid investigation in the diagnostic workup of scleroderma-spectrum disorders and, tellingly, was included in the most recent ACR/EULAR systemic sclerosis classification criteria [4]. As a consequence, there has never been more interest in capillaroscopy and contemporary research is actively evaluating both the additional utility of NFC within scleroderma-spectrum disorders as well as in other diseases characterised by microvasculopathy. This chapter will summarise the techniques and principles of NFC, its established role, and explore the emerging roles for NFC with a focus on connective-tissue diseases.

2. What is nailfold capillaroscopy?

As the name implies, NFC involves visualising the nailfold capillaries. Capillaries are the smallest blood vessels, with a size that normally allows the passage of a single red blood cell at a time. They form a complex network of "loops" (U-shaped structures commonly compared to hairpins) with an afferent (arterial) and efferent (venous) limb and an apex connecting the two (see **Figure 1**). These small vessels aid the diffusion of gases and the movement of substrates for and non-essential by-products of cellular respiration. The skin has a rich network of capillaries which are usually orientated vertically, distributing blood from the deep cutaneous arterioles to the surface skin and then back down again to the venous plexus. In contrast, at the nailfolds, these capillary loops lie horizontally which allows a visualisation along the length of their course. To be strictly accurate, we are not able to visualise the capillaries themselves, the thin walls of which are essentially transparent, but instead the column of red blood cells. Over many years researchers have identified abnormalities in the structure and arrangement of these capillaries present in certain diseases characterised by microvasculopathy. These abnormalities are discussed in more detail later.

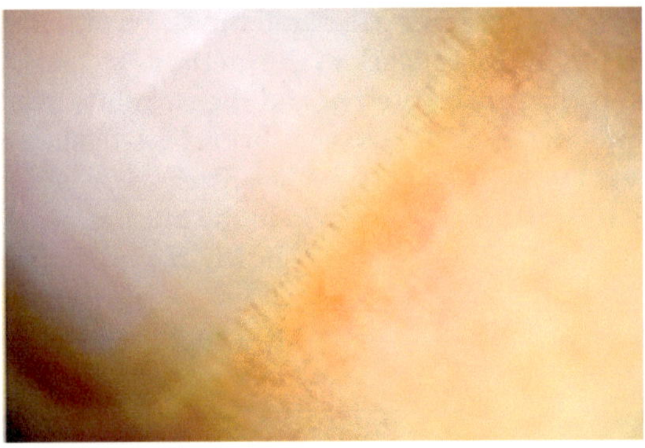

Figure 1.
Normal nailfold capillaries. The typical appearance of capillary "loops".

3. Nailfold capillaroscopy techniques

NFC consists of two interrelated elements, image acquisition and image interpretation, and these will be discussed in turn in this and the following sections.

3.1 General principles

For all techniques, there are a number of general principles that should be observed. Firstly, to minimise the potential for variability in findings due to vasoconstriction and altered digital perfusion, capillaroscopy should be performed in a warm environment, with most studies suggesting a 15–30 minute period of acclimatisation to "room temperature", usually around 20°C. Subjects should be advised to avoid smoking, caffeine or medications (where possible) that could cause peripheral vasoconstriction immediately prior to the investigation. Secondly, visualisation of the nailfold capillaries is aided by the use of a gel or oil interface to reduce surface reflection from the device light source. The more commonly used substances are clear or lightly coloured oils (such as paraffin or light olive oil) or lubricant jellies, applied in the region of the nailbed and cuticle immediately prior to visualisation. There are an increasing number of differing techniques for acquiring images and we will discuss the most frequently employed.

3.2 Widefield stereomicroscopy

Widefield stereomicroscopy (WSM; see **Figure 2a**) is the original technique pioneered by Maricq et al. and is still considered one of the two "gold-standard" techniques [2, 3, 5]. Each nailfold (usually of just the index-little finger of each hand, as thumbs can be difficult to orientate under the microscope) is examined at around 20-fold magnification which allows for a panoramic view of the entire nailfold. The microscope allows close control of depth of focus. The microscope can be combined with a camera and other digital equipment to allow recording of images and assist real-time explanation of investigation findings. The technique typically takes around 5 minutes to complete.

3.3 High-magnification videocapillaroscopy

Nailfold videocapillaroscopy (NVC; see **Figure 2b**) is the other "gold-standard" technique and is now the most frequent technique used in capillaroscopy research. Either a fixed or handheld imaging device is used which, when combined with computer software, affords a highly magnified view of the nailfold at 200–300-fold. This technique allows for very detailed images but an important consequence is that not all the nailfold can be visualised at the same time. The impact of this can be particularly relevant to studies looking at longitudinal nailfold changes (see later), as it can be difficult at subsequent study visits to visualise the exact same region of the nailfold. There is software that can 'stitch' together images using digital picture recognition and therefore produce a panoramic nailfold image made up of smaller high magnification images, first used by Herrick et al., which can mitigate this issue [6]. NVC can take substantially longer than other techniques if all fingers are studied (20–30 minutes), and consequently many studies restrict image acquisition to a single finger in both hands (most commonly the ring finger). An important potential downside of this compromise is that nailfold changes can vary markedly between even adjacent fingers. NVC has been shown in multiple studies to have good intra- and inter-observer variability and/or concordance and correlates well with WSM [6–9].

3.4 Handheld devices—ophthalmoscopes, dermatoscopes, USB microscopes etc.

Two important factors that have limited accessibility to NFC and its use in the broader rheumatology community are the relative (expensive) cost and the lack of portability of the two gold-standard techniques. There are clear advantages to being able to take a test to the "bedside" rather than having to bring a patient to the test, which is often only currently available at a small number of specialist institutions. Fortuitously, there are a number of low cost and handheld devices such as dermatoscopes and ophthalmoscopes which achieve a good visualisation of the nailfolds at around 10–20-fold magnification (see **Figure 2c**). A number of studies directly comparing these techniques with WSM and NVC have found a reassuring concordance [10–12]. In particular, although the rate of "unclassifiable" images is higher, ample diagnostically relevant findings can be elicited, even if more subtle changes can be missed. Rapidly improving technology, particularly with the availability of USB microscopes or attachments for smartphones, can already achieve similar magnification to NVC and record images. This infers that these devices are going to become more commonplace [11]. An additional advantage with the handheld devices is that they can be easier to use in patients with finger deformities and in thumbs (or even toes) which are often not visualised in other techniques, although the additional information gleaned from these is not yet of clear clinical utility.

4. Nailfold capillary abnormalities

Before proceeding to discuss nailfold capillary abnormalities, it is important to note that there is a surprisingly broad range of capillary appearances between or even within 'normal' subjects and the disease controls used in research settings [13]. It can sometimes be difficult to be certain whether subtle changes are of significance or not but with increasing experience this distinction becomes somewhat easier. In practice, most examinations will clearly fall into a normal or definitely abnormal category and for those that do not there is usually extra information from a history, examination and additional diagnostic tests that can help contextualise the capillaroscopy results.

The abnormal features that originally defined Maricq's "scleroderma-dermatomyositis pattern (SD-pattern) remain the most important to examine for [2]. These consist of giant (significantly enlarged) capillaries, avascular areas (also referred to as capillary "drop-out"), and microhaemorrhages. Other abnormalities are recognised and include excessively tortuous capillaries, unusually shaped capillaries ("bushy" or "arborized" capillaries) and cuticular hypertrophy, but their clinical significance especially in isolation is less well established.

4.1 Giant capillaries

There is no universally agreed definition of a "giant capillary" but one is by and large accepted as a capillary that is that is enlarged over four-fold normal diameter (and often >ten-fold) (see **Figure 3**). A normal adult capillary is somewhere between 25-50um and therefore generally anything over 150um is considered pathologic. Enlarged capillaries are somewhere in between giant capillaries and normal. A useful clinical tip is to compare capillaries within the same patient to first establish the appearances and dimensions of their "normal" capillaries and use these to compare the enlarged capillaries against, if present. The presence of even a single giant capillary is very suggestive of an underlying connective tissue disease.

4.2 Avascular areas

Avascular areas or areas of capillary "drop-out" are regions where there are no capillaries and in the absence of local nailfold trauma are highly specific for

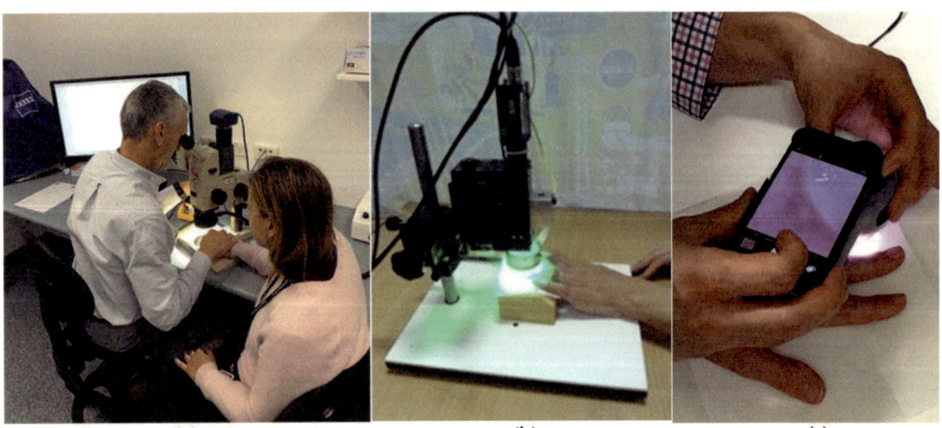

(a) (b) (c)

Figure 2.
The different techniques for performing nailfold capillaroscopy. (a) Widefield microscopy; (b) videocapillaroscopy; (c) dermoscopy (with a smartphone attachment).

systemic sclerosis in particular (see **Figure 4**). Again, there is no internationally ratified definition but a working definition is a 1 mm region of the distal nailfold with no capillaries present. Another definition is the absence of two or more sequential capillary loops [14]. It can be difficult if there is not adequate visualisation of the nailfold for technical reasons or if it is difficult to get the appropriate depth of focus to bring all capillaries in to view. A simple tip is to compare within the same patients nailfolds to see if the usual density of capillaries (number within a defined width or area) is regionally varied.

4.3 Microhaemorrhages

These are evidenced by reddish-brown punctate lesions (haemosiderin staining) in the cuticle (see **Figure 5**). They are often associated with regional capillary architectural abnormalities (such as a giant capillary) and sometimes recurrent haemorrhage can be deduced from lesions "growing-out" along the cuticle over time.

4.4 Other abnormal capillary shapes

It is difficult to define "bushy", "arborized" or excessively tortuous capillaries as these are qualitative judgements and experience dependent (see **Figure 6**). In addition, although cuticle hypertrophy is well recognised (although not that prevalent) there is no established definition for it and it is based upon a subjective assessment.

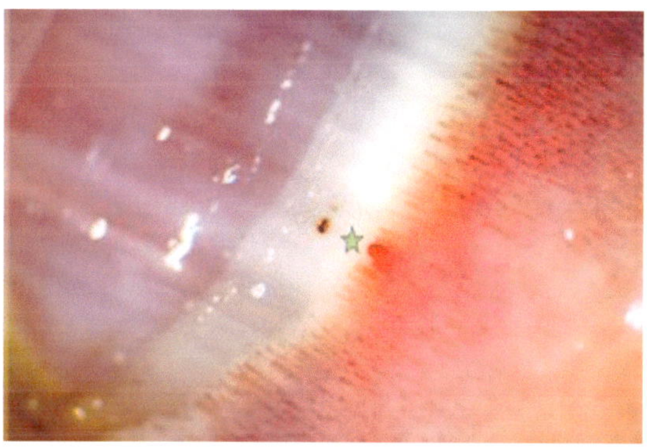

Figure 3.
A single giant capillary, in this example associated with a microhaemorrhage in the distal cuticle.

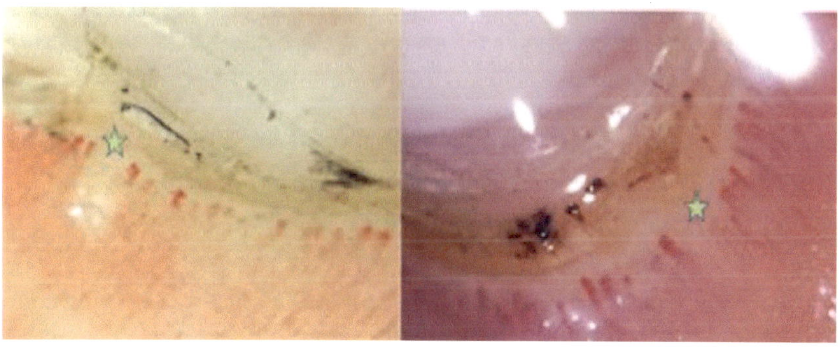

Figure 4.
Avascular areas, demonstrating areas of capillary "drop-out". Note in the right-hand image the extensive associated microhaemorrhages and cuticle hypertrophy.

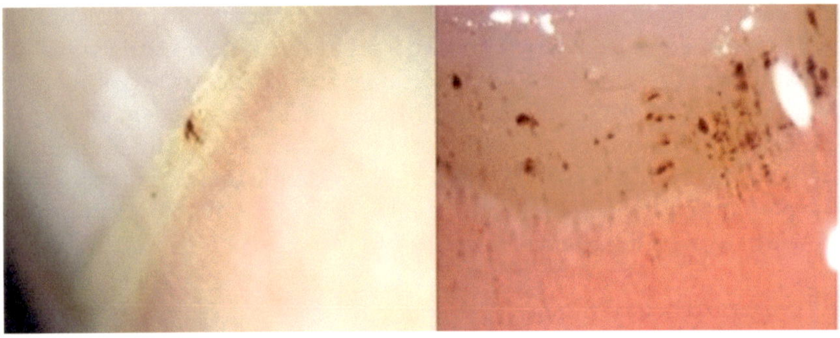

Figure 5.
Nailfold microhaemorrhages.

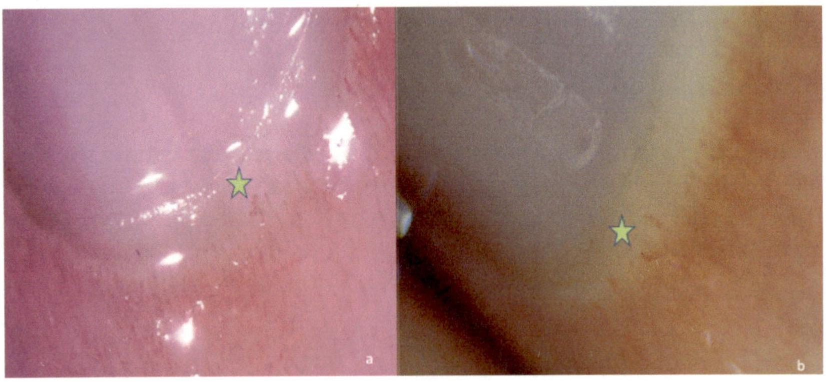

Figure 6.
Other abnormal capillary shapes. (a) A tortuous capillary; (b) elongated capillaries.

Recently, the reliability of simple capillaroscopic definitions to describe the different morphologies that can be seen in rheumatic diseases has been published and widely accepted [15]. Although there are a range of potential abnormalities which may seem relatively complex, there is actually very good intra- and inter-observer concordance in most studies and even only a short amount of training (for example an hour) can help complete novices make accurate assessments [16]. There has been encouraging results when capillaroscopy has been used in a primary care setting as well [17]. Two prospective studies in particular have elegantly demonstrated the prognostic significance of these abnormalities in patients with Raynaud's phenomenon. Koenig et al. showed that giant capillaries and capillary loss strongly predict the evolution to a diagnosis of systemic sclerosis (then using the 1980 ACR criteria) and, when combined with a relevant positive autoantibody, had a positive predictive value of 79% and negative predictive value of 93% [18]. A second study, by Ingegnoli et al., found that the three capillary abnormalities that correlated with a later diagnosis of systemic sclerosis were giant capillaries, capillary density and microhaemorrhages [19].

5. Classification

There is no universally adopted consensus on exactly how the varying combination of above potential capillary abnormalities should be classified and this is an ongoing research priority. Classification criteria have many discrete purposes from diagnostic criteria and we will cover only a few illustrative examples as our intended focus is on the use of capillaroscopy in the clinical rather than research setting.

5.1 Qualitative criteria

The first proposed classification criteria was that of Maricq et al. who classified patient's nailfold capillaries as having either "normal" appearances, "non-specific" abnormalities or the "Scleroderma-Dermatomyositis (or SD-) pattern" [2, 5]. This latter category was defined by the presence of giant capillaries or avascular areas and could include the other capillary abnormalities described above. It is this pattern that has now been shown in numerous publications to help differentiate primary from secondary Raynaud's syndrome and as the pattern present in around 90% of systemic sclerosis patients, often very early in the course of their disease [20]. In essence, therefore, it is these features that are of primary clinical significance as they strongly suggest an associated underlying connective-tissue disease. The "non-specific" group consists of individuals who have some definite capillary abnormalities (such as microhaemorrhages, enlarged or tortuous capillaries), but neither of the more specific features of giant capillaries or avascular areas. From a clinical perspective, the significance of an investigation with these findings should usually be interpreted as normal but it may have some suggestive relevance when considered in the context of a patient's history, examination and other investigations as supportive of a scleroderma-spectrum disorder.

5.2 Semi-quantitative criteria

Because of the intrinsic issues with purely qualitative classification systems, especially when trying to compare or reproduce different study methodologies and research findings, there have been many efforts to develop a more structured and systematic approach into criteria. A Brazilian group developed the Maricq scoring system and incorporated a count of the total number of enlarged or giant capillaries as well as a measure of mean capillary density (capillaries per mm) [21]. Other early efforts at moving towards a more quantitative classification included those by the research group of Lee et al. [14]. More recently, the most widely adopted criteria is that of Cutolo et al. who described "early", "active" and "late" categories (see **Table 1**) for individuals with definite capillary abnormal features [23]. Several studies have shown that the Cutolo criteria are associated with disease activity and severity. The "early" and "active" patterns are more common in limited SSc, whereas the "late" category is present more frequently in patients with diffuse SSc [24]. In the same study, the severity of organ involvement progressively increased across groups from "early" towards "late". Other studies have reported the "late" pattern in older patients, in those with a longer disease duration, and in those with diffuse disease [15, 16]. Several studies have shown that the "late" pattern in particular predicts digital ulcers as well as more severe cutaneous, cardiac and pulmonary disease [21–27]. The initial Cutolo criteria was later simplified into a score ranging from 0 to 9, correlating to the average score for each of three variables in each of eight examined nailfolds [28].

Classification	Description
Early	Few giant capillaries, few haemorrhages and no capillary loss
Active	Numerous giant capillaries and microhaemorrhages, mild capillary architecture disturbance and moderate capillary loss
Late	Severe capillary loss with extensive avascular areas, disorganised capillaries and ramified capillaries.

Table 1.
The Cutolo classification criteria [22].

5.3 Quantitative criteria

Certain components of the capillaroscopic assessment are well suited to quantitative assessment. Capillary density (by convention the number of capillaries within a 1 mm region of the distal nailfold) is the best example of this, with anything less than 6 per mm being pathologically abnormal. A quantitative method was employed in a recent multicentre study and involved counting all the microhaemorrhages, normal capillaries, enlarged capillaries, giant capillaries and other abnormal capillary shapes in the distal row within two 1 mm fields per finger [29]. The study concluded that the simple count of capillaries (i.e. capillary density) was sufficient to monitor the progression of scleroderma. Recently, some groups have used computer technology to count capillaries and automate this quantitative process with good reproducibility and obvious potential advantages for future work [30, 31]. Reduced capillary density has been associated with disease complications such as pulmonary hypertension, interstitial lung disease and digital ulcers. Many other capillary features have been measured and investigated including, for example, capillary length, angle and loop diameter, but the clinical relevance of these measurements is not well established.

6. The established role

6.1 Distinguishing primary from secondary Raynaud's syndrome

The first clearly established clinically relevant role for capillaroscopy was in the assessment of patients with Raynaud's symptoms. Abnormal nailfold capillaroscopy is strongly predictive of an underlying connective tissue disease (synonymous with "secondary" Raynaud's syndrome) and, conversely, normal nailfold capillaroscopy is reassuring that an underlying connective tissue disease is unlikely ("primary" Raynaud's syndrome). The early work into the importance of nailfold capillary changes in identifying patients with secondary Raynaud's syndrome is well summarised in a systematic review from 1998, where abnormal capillaries had the highest odds ratio (OR) of any variable studied for progression to secondary diseases [32]. These findings have been replicated and enhanced in the prospective study of Koenig et al. over 3000 patient years, who found abnormal capillaries and systemic sclerosis-specific autoantibodies were both independent predictors of an underlying connective tissue disease [18]. Twenty-six percent of patients with capillary abnormalities at baseline (and 36% with a specific autoantibody) developed systemic sclerosis within follow up, which increased to 80% in subjects with both features. Conversely, only 1.8% of patients with neither present at baseline developed a connective tissue disease during follow up. Similarly, a study from Pavlov-Dolijanovic et al. found 45% of their 3029 consecutive patients with Raynaud's syndrome and abnormal NFC went on to develop a connective tissue disease. The OR for being diagnosed with systemic sclerosis in patients with abnormal NFC compared to those with Raynaud's syndrome without capillary abnormalities was 183 (95% confidence intervals 97.9–271.5) [33].

6.2 Diagnosing systemic sclerosis

Abnormal capillaroscopy features are particularly useful in the diagnosis of systemic sclerosis (SSc) and are present in up to 90% of patients [34]. The work of Leroy and Medsger highlighted the importance of NFC in detecting early SSc in particular and much subsequent work has helped include capillaroscopy in the most recent SSc classification criteria (see **Table 2**) [4, 35]. Abnormal capillaroscopic findings contribute 2 points towards the 9 points necessary to establish a diagnosis of SSc. If combined with Raynaud's symptoms, a common indication for the investigation, it contributes a total of 4 points towards the diagnosis. The addition of capillaroscopy to the new criteria have helped improve their sensitivity for early and very early SSc which is an area of great interest to researchers seeking to find interventions and treatments to improve long-term outcomes [36, 37]. It could be argued on the basis of these criteria that access to NFC should be a pre-requisite for all clinicians and researchers evaluating patients with potential SSc.

6.3 A predictor of organ-specific manifestations in systemic sclerosis

There is an accumulating literature on the association between capillaroscopic findings and certain organ-specific complications of SSc. In general, the more severe morphological changes correlate with more severe disease [34, 38]. The converse is also true, where patients with less marked NFC abnormalities have less severe cutaneous and pulmonary involvement [39].

6.3.1 Digital ulcers

Digital ulcers (DU) are a visible representation of peripheral vasculopathy, occurring in up to 50% of patients at some point in their illness [40]. It stands to reason that capillaroscopic abnormalities would correlate with their presence and there has been considerable interest in applying capillaroscopy as a predictor of digital ulcers in systemic sclerosis. The association of capillary loss and digital ischaemia was first established almost a decade ago with work by Herrick et al. and Ennis et al. [37, 41]. The more recent video CAPillaroscopy (CAP) study showed the

Item	Sub-item	Weight/score
Skin thickening of fingers of both hands extending proximal to the MCPs	–	9
Skin thickening (only count the higher score)	Puffy fingers	2
	Sclerodactyly	4
Finger tip lesions (only count the higher score)	Digital tip ulcers	2
	Finger tip pitting scars	3
Telangiectasia	–	2
Abnormal nailfolds	–	2
Pulmonary arterial hypertension and/or interstitial lung disease (maximum of 2)	Pulmonary arterial hypertension	2
	Interstitial lung disease	2
Raynaud's phenomenon	–	2
SSc-related autoantibodies (maximum score is 3)	Anti-Scl70 (anti-topoisomerase I)	3
	Anti-centromere	
	Anti-RNA polymerase III	

Patients with a score of ≥9 are classified as having definite systemic sclerosis.

Table 2.
The 2013 classification criteria for systemic sclerosis [4].

mean number of capillaries in the dominant hand middle finger (per mm) was one of three predictors of DU (the two others being number of DUs at enrolment and critical digital ischaemia at enrolment) [29]. The "late" NFC pattern (see **Table 1**) has been shown in a prospective longitudinal study to be an independent predictor for DU in patients both with and without a history of DUs [42]. NFC findings may help in future target high risk patients for vascular remodelling and protective strategies. Indeed, a prognostic tool, the capillaroscopic skin ulcer risk index (CSURI), has been developed and demonstrated to help predict ulcers in the 3 months following assessment [43]. Another similar tool to predict digital trophic lesions intended for day-to-day clinical used based upon a simple capillary count has also been described [44].

6.3.2 Pulmonary hypertension

Pulmonary hypertension affects around 15% of patients with systemic sclerosis and despite advances in therapy still accounts for substantial morbidity and mortality [45]. Because of its relatively lower prevalence than other organ specific manifestations, it is more difficult to explore the role of NFC in predicting its presence or severity but some studies have already shown some intriguing results. In a recent Dutch cohort of over 200 patients, NFC changes were independently predictive of cardio-respiratory complications and, notably, all patients with pulmonary hypertension had abnormal NFC [46]. The "late" pattern and reduced capillary density have both been associated with the presence and severity of pulmonary hypertension in SSc [47, 48].

6.3.3 Interstitial lung disease

Interstitial lung disease (ILD) is present in up to 80% of patients with systemic sclerosis and, although only around 25% develop progressive disease, this again contributes to substantial morbidity and mortality [35]. In a retrospective observational study an association was found between abnormal NFC and the presence of ILD [49]. Capillaroscopic abnormalities were associated with a mean 15% reduction in forced vital capacity and DLCO compared to participants with normal capillaroscopy findings. Multiple other studies have also found an association between abnormal capillaroscopy and the presence or severity of ILD [27, 34, 46].

6.3.4 Mortality

Abnormal NFC has been associated with an increased mortality. A study of almost 3000 patients with Raynaud's symptoms but without an established diagnosis of a CTD was conducted for a mean of 9.3 years. An increased all-cause mortality rate was found for females (HR 1.10; 1.07–1.77) but this association was interestingly not found for males, although the substantially fewer males with Raynaud's syndrome and relatively short follow up for this outcome measure may have impacted [50]. A more recent study also found an association between capillary loss and mortality, although this did not remain significant after multi-variant adjustment [51].

7. The emerging role

There has never been more activity and interest in capillaroscopy and its applications are only likely to expand over time. Although its role in the diagnosis of SSc is well established, it is emerging as having a role in a variety of other CTDs such as the idiopathic inflammatory myopathies (IIM) and mixed connective tissue disease (MCTD). Even within SSc there is much ongoing work into further understanding the potential role for capillaroscopy in more accurately screening and monitoring for disease complications and as a putative biomarker. Others are evaluating the potential role of capillaroscopy in monitoring the efficacy of new therapies and as a trial outcome measure. Finally, it is likely that capillaroscopy can be combined with complementary technologies or investigations to better serve the need for progress in the understanding and management of CTDs.

7.1 Use in other connective tissue diseases

7.1.1 Idiopathic inflammatory myopathies

Implicit in Maricq's initial qualitative classification of the "scleroderma-dermatomyositis" pattern was a recognition that dermatomyositis (DM) had similar nailfold capillary changes to SSc. This perhaps is not surprising given, like SSc, DM is a condition characterised by microvasculopathy and, along with other IIM subtypes such as the anti-synthetase syndrome and overlap myositis, it shares many clinical manifestations such as Raynaud's syndrome, myositis and cutaneous involvement [52]. NFC has not been as thoroughly evaluated in this patient group as in SSc but there are some interesting findings. An Italian study of 52 patients with IIM found nailfold changes were significantly more common in patients with DM versus polymyositis (PM) and that disease duration seemed to have an impact on the features, as patients with longer disease duration had less of the "late" features [53]. This may seem counter-intuitive and the opposite of the findings in SSc where there is a trend towards more "late" pattern changes with increasing disease duration, but the study was not controlled for the impact of treatment on the capillary features. In an earlier study from Spain, the combination of microhaemorrhages and capillary enlargement was found more frequently in patients with DM *versus* PM (OR 8.9) and overall in their cohort of 53 patients with IIM, found the prevalence of abnormal NFC to be 43% [54]. This study also found an association between NFC abnormalities and both disease activity and damage. There was a low incidence of capillary loss (in 20% of DM patients and 0% of PM patients) and the authors concluded that the pathogenesis of the disease is therefore likely different from that of systemic sclerosis, where avascular areas are far more prominent. The authors also concluded that abnormal NFC contributed to an earlier diagnosis of IIM and likely marks out patients for a poorer prognosis. There is limited information on longitudinal changes over time in patients with IIM but one study of quantitative capillaroscopy in these patients *versus* healthy controls found a progressive reduction in capillary density in patients with anti-Jo-1 positive anti-synthetase syndrome [55]. Another recent study has reported some relatively subtle longitudinal differences in the nailfolds of patients with IIM compared to SSc [56].

7.1.2 Mixed connective tissue disease

Many patients with MCTD, which again shares considerable clinical manifestation overlap with SSc, will have NFC abnormalities although this has not been studied in isolation [33]. The recent study by Markusse et al. found that the "early" pattern was associated with a positive anti-RNP antibody, a hint that, similar to NFC in the IIM, MCTD may have differing underlying microvascular pathophysiology with less avascular areas or capillary drop-out compared to patients with SSc [46].

7.1.3 Systemic lupus erythematosus

In a recent systematic review, Cutolo et al. have helped summarise the limited existing literature of NFC in systemic lupus erythematosus (SLE) [57]. Although differences in the prevalence of capillary abnormalities in patients with SLE compared to normal controls have been found (especially with increased capillary tortuosity, prominent venous plexus and elongated capillaries), these are usually subtle compared to the more marked findings in SSc and IIM. An increased NFC score did correlate with disease activity in the majority of the few studies that reported on this, especially with the frequency of Raynaud's symptoms or digital gangrene.

7.2 Capillaroscopy as a putative biomarker

Although the role of NFC in diagnosis is well established, its role, if any, in established disease is less clear – could serial examinations be used to screen for complications in much the same way as an annual echocardiogram and pulmonary function tests would do? Prospective longitudinal studies are required to properly address this question, and some are already completed or underway. A recent study by Avouac et al. followed patients prospectively over three years and found that changes in NFC over time (in particular a loss of capillary density to <4 per mm), which occurred in almost half of patients, was a strong marker of organ progression [58]. As mentioned above numerous studies have linked the "late" NFC pattern with SSc disease activity, digital ulcers, cutaneous, cardiac and pulmonary involvement, which suggests an evolution of NFC changes over time [24, 26, 27]. A study from Brazil looked at overall mortality within a group of patients with SSc and found an increased mortality in those with more marked capillary loss [59]. Longitudinal NFC assessments in patients with systemic sclerosis could become feasibly become a part of routine care [60]. The comprehensive review by Ingegnoli & Gualtierotti also summarises the literature to date on the association between abnormalities of NFC and other serum biomarkers such as endothelin-1 and VEGF, which offers an insight into a potential future where biomarkers could be combined to stratify patients and personalise management [9].

7.3 Nailfold capillaroscopy and therapeutics

Another area that is being researched intensively is in the arena of monitoring effects of drugs on nailfold changes. If, as has been largely established, the structural microvascular changes in CTDs can associate with disease activity, it would also make sense that a successful treatment may reverse the microvascular changes. NFC could therefore be used as a measure of treatment efficacy or even a trial outcome measure. There have been reports of significant improvements in microangiopathy paralleling the substantial clinical improvement in patients after autologous haematopoeitic stem cell transplant (HSCT) for SSc as well as in a patient with anti-synthetase syndrome [61–63]. In one report (of two patients with SSc and MCTD respectively), progressive improvements in NFC were seen with the cyclophosphamide used for stem cell mobilisation and then the subsequent HSCT [63]. Despite the evidence that endothelin-1 inhibitors reduce the incidence of digital ulcer recurrence and Raynaud's symptoms [64–66], two studies have failed to find significant changes in structural microvascular changes [67, 68]. However, the follow up of these studies was relatively short and it has been argued that the true impact of endothelin-1 antagonists on structural microvascular change may take longer to establish. Similarly, intravenous prostanoid therapy was not associated with NFC improvements at 12 months despite a statistically significant improvement in Raynaud's symptoms [69]. Some researchers are already postulating that making an early diagnosis of SSc in patients with NFC abnormalities may allow for the early instigation of preventative therapies (e.g. endothelin-1 antagonists to prevent pulmonary hypertension, antifibrotic therapies to prevent ILD) and therefore help change the natural history of the disease [70].

7.4 Combining NFC with other technologies

As technology rapidly advances there may become available a variety of novel techniques that allow for image acquisition. Inexpensive USB microscopes are already available as are accessory equipment allowing the digital camera of a smart phone to take diagnostically useful images [11]. Technology could also be harnessed to allow for quicker and more reproducible image assessment, as in the case of the recent publication of automated capillary counting [30]. NFC is an excellent measure of structural microvascular changes in disease, but the role and assessment of functional changes may also add clinically useful information. Thermography, where the skin surface temperature is measured using thermal cameras, is already well established at some expert centres [20]. The equipment is relatively expensive and requires regular calibration but technology is advancing and soon thermal cameras may be available as smartphone attachments. Several studies have shown thermography to be able to differentiate between healthy controls and primary Raynaud's and between primary Raynaud's and Raynaud's secondary to systemic sclerosis based upon an abnormal pattern (a persistent "distal-dorsal difference") of rewarming [71, 72]. Although thermography as a stand-alone test has some utility, further work may help establish that, in time, assessments of patients with potential CTD may include both a structural assessment in the form of NFC and a functional assessment. Developing a standardised protocol for thermography with a plan to validate the protocol to assist ongoing research in thermography is already underway [39]. Another novel strategy for functional perfusion assessment is to use Laser technology. Techniques such as laser Doppler flowmetry and laser speckle contrast analysis (LASCA) have shown good reliability in patients with SSc [73–77]. Advances are occurring in parallel with advances in other non-invasive imaging techniques such as optical coherence tomography and photoacoustic imaging which allow the opportunity to view the skin and cutaneous vessels in three dimensions [20].

8. Future directions

Despite the great progress made by research into NFC over the last 50 years there is much work that is still required to be done. There is a great need for a widely accepted consensus classification criteria. Work needs to continue to improve awareness of and access to the investigation which will be aided by more convenient and cheaper technologies. Prospective longitudinal studies will allow for a better understanding of certain nailfold capillary abnormalities and their link with organ-specific complications, disease severity, disease activity and hopefully, in time, the efficacy of certain treatments. Further work will also target other related CTDs.

9. Conclusions

Nailfold capillaroscopy is a simple, non-invasive, and non-expensive investigation with established roles in the diagnosis of scleroderma-spectrum disorders as well as being linked to the presence and severity of a variety of serious organ-specific manifestations which account for substantial morbidity and mortality. Access to the investigation is likely to increase as technology makes equipment more user friendly, reproducible and inexpensive. Demand for the investigation is similarly going to increase substantially as it has been included in recent classification criteria for SSc and the potential clinical applications are only increasing in a wide range of conditions characterised by microangiopathy. Because microvascular change is often present very early in the clinical disease course, nailfold capillaroscopy may be a tool to identify a "window of opportunity", in conditions which to date have proven largely refractory to the therapies employed with much greater success in other rheumatic and autoimmune disease. It may usher in a new era of preventative rather than reactionary therapy and may become a part of disease management decisions, perhaps in a similar way to the use of clinical ultrasound in patients with rheumatoid arthritis. It is of relevance to all clinicians seeing patients with suspected connective tissue diseases to stay abreast of the progress being made in nailfold capillaroscopy and the related investigations.

Acknowledgements

The authors would like to thank the patients of Royal Prince Alfred Hospital.

Conflict of interests

The authors declare no conflict of interests.

Author details

Matthew J.S. Parker[1,2*] and Neil W. McGill[1,2]

1 Department of Rheumatology, Royal Prince Alfred Hospital, Sydney, NSW, Australia

2 University of Sydney, Sydney, NSW, Australia

*Address all correspondence to: mjsparker24@gmail.com

References

[1] Brown G, O'Leary P. Skin capillaries in scleroderma. Archives of Internal Medicine. 1926;**36**:73-88

[2] Maricq H, LeRoy E. Patterns of finger capillary abnormalities in connective tissue disease by "wide-field" microscopy. Arthritis and Rheumatism. 1973;**16**(5):619-628

[3] Maricq HR, LeRoy EC, D'Angelo WA, Medsger TA Jr, Rodnan GP, Sharp GCWJ. Diagnostic potential of in vivo capillary microscopy in scleroderma and related disorders. Arthritis and Rheumatism. 1980;**23**(2):183-189

[4] Van Den Hoogen F, Khanna D, Fransen J, Johnson SR, Baron M, Tyndall A, et al. 2013 Classification criteria for systemic sclerosis: An american college of rheumatology/European league against rheumatism collaborative initiative. Annals of the Rheumatic Diseases. 2013;**72**:1747-1755

[5] Maricq HR. Widefield capillary microscopy. Technique and rating scale for abnormalities seen in scleroderma and related disorders. Arthritis and Rheumatism. 1981;**24**(9):1159-1165

[6] Anderson ME, Allen PD, Moore T, Hillier V, Taylor CJ, Ariane L, et al. Computerized nailfold video capillaroscopy—A new tool for assessment of Raynaud's phenomenon. Journal of Rheumatology. 2005;**32**(5):841-848

[7] Sekiyama JY, Camargo CZ, Andrade LEC, Kayser C. Reliability of widefield nailfold capillaroscopy and videocapillaroscopy in the assessment of patients with Raynaud's phenomenon. Arthritis Care and Research. 2013;**65**(11):1853-1861

[8] Dinsdale G, Moore T, O'Leary N, Tresadern P, Berks M, Roberts C, et al. Intra-and inter-observer reliability of nailfold videocapillaroscopy—A possible outcome measure for systemic sclerosis-related microangiopathy. Microvascular Research. 2017;**112**:1-6

[9] Ingegnoli F, Gualtierotti R. A systematic overview on the use and relevance of capillaroscopy in systemic sclerosis. Expert Review of Clinical Immunology. 2013;**9**(11):1091-1097

[10] Hughes M, Moore T, O'Leary N, Tracey A, Ennis H, Dinsdale G, et al. A study comparing videocapillaroscopy and dermoscopy in the assessment of nailfold capillaries in patients with systemic sclerosis-spectrum disorders. Rheumatology (Oxford, England). 2015;**54**(8):1435-1442

[11] Parker MJS, Oliffe MT, McGill NW. An evaluation of two novel capillaroscopy techniques in suspected scleroderma-spectrum disorders: A single-Centre cross-sectional study. Modern Rheumatology. 2018;**28**(4):676-680

[12] Dogan S, Akdogan A, Atakan N. Nailfold capillaroscopy in systemic sclerosis: Is there any difference between videocapillaroscopy and dermatoscopy? Skin Research and Technology. 2013;**19**(4):446-449

[13] Ingegnoli F, Gualtierotti R, Lubatti C, Bertolazzi C, Gutierrez M, Boracchi P, et al. Nailfold capillary patterns in healthy subjects: A real issue in capillaroscopy. Microvascular Research. 2013;**90**:90-95

[14] Lee P, Leung F, Alderdice C, Armstrong S. Nailfold capillary microscopy in the connective tissue diseases: A semi-quantitative assessment. The Journal of Rheumatology. 1983;**10**(6):930-938

[15] Cutolo M, Melsens K, Herrick AL, Foeldvari I, Deschepper E,

De Keyser F, et al. Reliability of simple capillaroscopic definitions in describing capillary morphology in rheumatic diseases. Rheumatology (United Kingdom). 2018;**57**(4):757-759

[16] Smith V, Beeckman S, Herrick AL, Decuman S, Deschepper E, De Keyser F, et al. An EULAR study group pilot study on reliability of simple capillaroscopic definitions to describe capillary morphology in rheumatic diseases. Rheumatology (Oxford, England). 2016;**55**(5):883-890

[17] Overbury R, Murtaugh MA, Fischer A, Frech TM. Primary care assessment of capillaroscopy abnormalities in patients with Raynauds phenomenon. Clinical Rheumatology. 2015;**34**(12):2135-2140

[18] Koenig M, Joyal F, Fritzler MJ, Roussin A, Abrahamowicz M, Boire G, et al. Autoantibodies and microvascular damage are independent predictive factors for the progression of Raynaud's phenomenon to systemic sclerosis: A twenty-year prospective study of 586 patients, with validation of proposed criteria for early systemic sclerosi. Arthritis and Rheumatism. 2008;**58**(12):3902-3912

[19] Ingegnoli F, Boracchi P, Gualtierotti R, Lubatti C, Meani L, Zahalkova L, et al. Prognostic model based on nailfold capillaroscopy for identifying Raynaud's phenomenon patients at high risk for the development of a scleroderma spectrum disorder: PRINCE (Prognostic Index for Nailfold Capillaroscopic Examination). Arthritis and Rheumatism. 2008;**58**(7):2174-2182

[20] Herrick AL, Murray A. The role of capillaroscopy and thermography in the assessment and management of Raynaud's phenomenon. Autoimmunity Reviews. 2018;**17**(5):465-472

[21] Correa MJU, Andrade LEC, Kayser C. Comparison of laser Doppler imaging, fingertip lacticemy test, and nailfold capillaroscopy for assessment of digital microcirculation in systemic sclerosis. Arthritis Research & Therapy. 2010;**12**:R157

[22] Cutolo M, Sulli A, Pizzorni C, Accardo S. Nailfold capillaroscopy assessment of microvascular damage in systemic sclerosis. The Journal of Rheumatology. 2000;**27**:155-160

[23] Cutolo M, Pizzorni C, Tuccio M, Burroni A, Craviotto C, Basso M, et al. Nailfold videocapillaroscopic patterns and serum autoantibodies in systemic sclerosis. Rheumatology. 2004;**43**(6):719-726

[24] Caramaschi P, Canestrini S, Martinelli N, Volpe A, Pieropan S, Ferrari M, et al. Scleroderma patients nailfold videocapillaroscopic patterns are associated with disease subset and disease severity. Rheumatology. 2007;**46**(10):1566-1569

[25] Marino Claveri L, Knobel E, Takashima L, Techera L, Oliver M, Gonzalez P, et al. Organ involvement in Argentinian systemic sclerosis patients with "late" pattern as compared to patients with "early/active" pattern by nailfold capillaroscopy. Clinical Rheumatology. 2013;**32**(6):839-843

[26] Smith V, Decuman S, Sulli A, Bonroy C, Piettte Y, Deschepper E, et al. Do worsening scleroderma capillaroscopic patterns predict future severe organ involvement? A pilot study. Annals of the Rheumatic Diseases. 2012;**71**(10):1636-1639

[27] Smith V, Riccieri V, Pizzorni C, Decuman S, Deschepper E, Bonroy C, et al. Nailfold capillaroscopy for prediction of novel future severe organ involvement in systemic sclerosis. The Journal of Rheumatology. 2013;**40**(12):2023-2028

[28] Sulli A, Secchi ME, C Pizzorni MC. Scoring the nailfold microvascular changes during the capillaroscopic analysis in systemic sclerosis patients. Annals of the Rheumatic Diseases. 2008;**67**(6):885-887

[29] Cutolo M, Herrick AL, Distler O, Becker MO, Beltran E, Carpentier P, et al. Nailfold Videocapillaroscopic features and other clinical risk factors for digital ulcers in systemic sclerosis: A multicenter, prospective cohort study. Arthritis Rheumatol. 2016;**68**(10):2527-2539

[30] Cheng C, Lee CW, Daskalakis C. A reproducible computerized method for quantitation of capillary density using nailfold capillaroscopy. Journal of Visualized Experiments. 2015;**104**:1-8

[31] Cutolo M, Trombetta AC, Melsens K, Pizzorni C, Sulli A, Ruaro B, et al. Automated assessment of absolute nailfold capillary number on videocapillaroscopic images: Proof of principle and validation in systemic sclerosis. Microcirculation. 2018;**25**(4):16-18

[32] Spencer-Green G. Outcomes in primary Raynaud phenomenon. Archives of Internal Medicine. 1998;**158**:595-600

[33] Pavlov-Dolijanovic S, Damjanov NS, Stojanovic RM, Vujasinovic Stupar NZ, Stanisavljevic DM. Scleroderma pattern of nailfold capillary changes as predictive value for the development of a connective tissue disease: A follow-up study of 3029 patients with primary Raynaud's phenomenon. Rheumatology International. 2012;**32**(10):3039-3045

[34] Ghizzoni C, Sebastiani M, Manfredi A, Campomori F, Colaci M, Giuggioli D, et al. Prevalence and evolution of scleroderma pattern at nailfold videocapillaroscopy in systemic sclerosis patients: Clinical and prognostic implications. Microvascular Research. 2015;**99**:92-95

[35] Khanna D, Nagaraja V, Tseng C hong, Abtin F, Suh R, Kim G, et al. Predictors of lung function decline in scleroderma-related interstitial lung disease based on high-resolution computed tomography: Implications for cohort enrichment in systemic sclerosis-associated interstitial lung disease trials. Arthritis Research & Therapy. 2015;**17**(1):1-10

[36] Jordan S, Maurer B, Toniolo M, Michel B, Distler O. Performance of the new ACR/EULAR classification criteria for systemic sclerosis in clinical practice. Rheumatology (Oxford, England). 2015;**54**(8):1454-1458

[37] Cutolo M, Smith V, Distler O, Kowal-Bielecka O, Allanore Y, Matucci-Cerinic M. OP0035 preliminary analysis of nailfold capillaroscopy in the very early diagnosis of systemic sclerosis (VEDOSS): The capi-vedoss experience. Annals of the Rheumatic Diseases. 2017;**76**:65-66

[38] Fichel F, Baudot N, Gaitz JP, Trad S, Barbe C, Francès C, et al. Systemic sclerosis with normal or nonspecific nailfold capillaroscopy. Dermatology. 2014;**228**(4):360-367

[39] Vayssairat M, Hidouche D, Abdoucheli-Baudot N, Gaitz JP. Clinical significance of subcutaneous calcinosis in patients with systemic sclerosis. Does diltiazem induce its regression? Annals of the Rheumatic Diseases. 1998;**57**(4):252-254

[40] Walker UA, Tyndall A, Czirják L, Denton C, Farge-Bancel D, Kowal-Bielecka O, et al. Clinical risk assessment of organ manifestations in systemic sclerosis: A report from the EULAR scleroderma trials and research group database. Annals of the Rheumatic Diseases. 2007;**66**(6):754-763

[41] Ennis H, Moore T, Murray A, Vail A, Herrick AL. Further confirmation that digital ulcers are associated with the severity of abnormality on nailfold capillaroscopy in patients with systemic sclerosis. Rheumatology (United Kingdom). 2014;**53**(2):376-377

[42] Silva I, Teixeira A, Oliveira J, Almeida I, Almeida R, Águas A, et al. Endothelial dysfunction and nailfold videocapillaroscopy pattern as predictors of digital ulcers in systemic sclerosis: A cohort study and review of the literature. Clinical Reviews in Allergy and Immunology. 2015;**49**(2):240-252

[43] Sebastiani M, Manfredi A, Colaci M, Damico R, Malagoli V, Giuggioli D, et al. Capillaroscopic skin ulcer risk index: A new prognostic tool for digital skin ulcer development in systemic sclerosis patients. Arthritis Care and Research. 2009;**61**(5):688-694

[44] Smith V, De Keyser F, Pizzorni C, Van Praet ET, Decuman S, Sulli A, et al. Nailfold capillaroscopy for day-to-day clinical use: Construction of a simple scoring modality as a clinical prognostic index for digital trophic lesions. Annals of the Rheumatic Diseases. 2011;**70**(1):180-183

[45] Denton CP, Khanna D. Systemic sclerosis. Lancet. 2017;**6736**(17):1-15

[46] Markusse IM, Meijs J, De BB, Bakker JA, Schippers HPC, Schouffoer AA, et al. Predicting cardiopulmonary involvement in patients with systemic sclerosis: Complementary value of nailfold videocapillaroscopy patterns and disease-specific autoantibodies. Rheumatology. 2017;**56**:1081-1088

[47] Hofstee HMA, Serné EH, Roberts C, Hesselstrand R, Scheja A, Moore TL, et al. A multicentre study on the reliability of qualitative and quantitative nail-fold videocapillaroscopy assessment. Rheumatology. 2012;**51**(4):749-755

[48] Riccieri V, Vasile M, Iannace N, Stefanantoni K, Sciarra I, Vizza CD, et al. Systemic sclerosis patients with and without pulmonary arterial hypertension: A nailfold capillaroscopy study. Rheumatology. 2013;**52**(8):1525-1528

[49] Castellví I, Simeón-Aznar CP, Sarmiento M, Fortuna A, Mayos M, Geli C, et al. Association between nailfold capillaroscopy findings and pulmonary function tests in patients with systemic sclerosis. The Journal of Rheumatology. 2015;**42**(2):222-227

[50] Mueller M, Gschwandtner ME, Gamper J, Giurgea GA, Charwat-Resl S, Kiener HP, et al. Relation of nailfold capillaries and autoantibodies to mortality in patients with raynaud phenomenon. Circulation. 2016;**133**(5):509-517

[51] Pavan TR, Bredemeier M, Hax V, Capobianco KG, da Silva Mendonça Chakr R, Xavier RM. Capillary loss on nailfold capillary microscopy is associated with mortality in systemic sclerosis. Clinical Rheumatology. 2018;**37**(2):475-481

[52] Parker MJS, Lilleker JB, Roberts ME, Chinoy H. Idiopathic inflammatory myopathies. Medicine (United Kingdom). 2018;**46**(2):140-145

[53] Manfredi A, Sebastiani M, Cassone G, Pipitone N, Giuggioli D, Colaci M, et al. Nailfold capillaroscopic changes in dermatomyositis and polymyositis. Clinical Rheumatology. 2015;**34**(2):279-284

[54] Selva-O'Callaghan A, Fonollosa-Pla V, Trallero-Araguás E, Martínez-Gómez X, Simeon-Aznar CP, Labrador-Horrillo M, et al. Nailfold capillary microscopy in adults with inflammatory myopathy.

Seminars in Arthritis and Rheumatism. 2010;**39**(5):398-404

[55] Mercer LK, Moore TL, Chinoy H, Murray AK, Vail A, Cooper RG, et al. Quantitative nailfold video capillaroscopy in patients with idiopathic inflammatory myopathy. Rheumatology. 2010;**49**(9):1699-1705

[56] Pizzorni C, Cutolo M, Sulli A, Ruaro B, Trombetta AC, Ferrari G, et al. Long-term follow-up of nailfold videocapillaroscopic changes in dermatomyositis versus systemic sclerosis patients. Clinical Rheumatology. 2018;**37**(10):2723-2729

[57] Cutolo M, Melsens K, Wijnant S, Ingegnoli F, Thevissen K, De Keyser F, et al. Nailfold capillaroscopy in systemic lupus erythematosus: A systematic review and critical appraisal. Autoimmunity Reviews. 2018;**17**(4):344-352

[58] Avouac J, Lepri G, Smith V, Toniolo E, Hurabielle C, Vallet A, et al. Sequential nailfold videocapillaroscopy examinations have responsiveness to detect organ progression in systemic sclerosis. Seminars in Arthritis and Rheumatism. 2017;**47**(1):86-94

[59] Kayser C, Sekiyama JY, Próspero LC, Camargo CZ, Andrade LEC, Próspero LC, et al. Nailfold capillaroscopy abnormalities as predictors of mortality in patients with systemic sclerosis. Clinical and Experimental Rheumatology. 2013;**31**:S103-S108

[60] Pauling JD. Could nailfold videocapillaroscopy usher in a new era of preventative disease-modifying therapeutic intervention in systemic sclerosis? Rheumatology. 2017;**56**(7):1053-1055

[61] Miniati I, Guiducci S, Conforti ML, Rogai V, Fiori G, Cinelli M, et al. Autologous stem cell transplantation improves microcirculation in systemic sclerosis. Annals of the Rheumatic Diseases. 2009;**68**(1):94-98

[62] Chojnowski MM, Nałęcz-Janik J. Regression of microangiopathy in antisynthetase syndrome. Rheumatology. 2017;**56**:724

[63] Aschwanden M, Daikeler T, Jaeger K, Thalhammer C, Gratwohl A, Matucci-Cerinic M, et al. Rapid improvement of nailfold capillaroscopy after intense immunosuppression for systemic sclerosis and mixed connective tissue disease. Annals of the Rheumatic Diseases. 2008;**67**(7):1057-1059

[64] Cutolo M, Zampogna G, Vremis L, Smith V, Pizzorni C, Sulli A. Longterm effects of endothelin receptor antagonism on microvascular damage evaluated by nailfold capillaroscopic analysis in systemic sclerosis. The Journal of Rheumatology. 2013;**40**(1):40-45

[65] Cutolo M, Ruaro B, Pizzorni C, Ravera F, Smith V, Zampogna G, et al. Longterm treatment with endothelin receptor antagonist bosentan and iloprost improves fingertip blood perfusion in systemic sclerosis. The Journal of Rheumatology. 2014;**41**(5):881-886

[66] Trombetta AC, Pizzorni C, Ruaro B, Paolino S, Sulli A, Smith V, et al. Effects of longterm treatment with bosentan and iloprost on nailfold absolute capillary number, fingertip blood perfusion, and clinical status in systemic sclerosis. The Journal of Rheumatology. 2016;**43**(11):2033-2041

[67] Hettema ME, Zhang D, Bootsma H, Kallenberg CGM. Bosentan therapy for patients with severe Raynaud's phenomenon in systemic sclerosis. Annals of the Rheumatic Diseases. 2007;**66**:1398-1399

[68] Moore TL, Vail A, Herrick AL. Assessment of digital vascular structure

and function in response to bosentan in patients with systemic sclerosis-related Raynaud's phenomenon (1). Rheumatology. 2007;**46**(2):363-364

[69] Shah P, Murray AK, Moore TL, Herrick AL. Effects of iloprost on microvascular structure assessed by nailfold videocapillaroscopy: A pilot study. Journal of Rheumatology. 2011;**38**(9):14-16

[70] Pauling JD. Could nailfold videocapillaroscopy usher in a new era of preventative disease-modifying therapeutic intervention in systemic sclerosis ? Rheumatology. 2017;**56**:1053-1055

[71] Anderson ME, Moore TL, Lunt M, Herrick AL. The "distal-dorsal difference": A thermographic parameter by which to differentiate between primary and secondary Raynaud's phenomenon. Rheumatology. 2007;**46**(3):533-538

[72] Horikoshi M, Inokuma S, Kijima Y, Kobuna M, Miura Y, Okada R, et al. Thermal disparity between fingers after cold-water immersion of hands: A useful Indicator of disturbed peripheral circulation in Raynaud phenomenon patients. Internal Medicine. 2016;**55**(5):461-466

[73] Lambrecht V, Cutolo M, De Keyser F, Decuman S, Ruaro B, Sulli A, et al. Reliability of the quantitative assessment of peripheral blood perfusion by laser speckle contrast analysis in a systemic sclerosis cohort. Annals of the Rheumatic Diseases. 2016;**75**(6):1263-1264

[74] Ruaro B, Sulli A, Pizzorni C, Paolino S, Smith V, Cutolo M. Correlations between skin blood perfusion values and nailfold capillaroscopy scores in systemic sclerosis patients. Microvascular Research. 2016;**105**:119-124

[75] Ruaro B, Sulli A, Alessandri E, Pizzorni C, Ferrari G, Cutolo M. Laser speckle contrast analysis: A new method to evaluate peripheral blood perfusion in systemic sclerosis patients. Annals of the Rheumatic Diseases. 2014;**73**(6):1181-1185

[76] Ruaro B, Sulli A, Pizzorni C, Paolino S, Smith V, Alessandri E, et al. Correlations between blood perfusion and dermal thickness in different skin areas of systemic sclerosis patients. Microvascular Research. 2018;**115**(8):28-33

[77] Cutolo M, Vanhaecke A, Ruaro B, Deschepper E, Ickinger C, Melsens K, et al. Is laser speckle contrast analysis (LASCA) the new kid on the block in systemic sclerosis? A systematic literature review and pilot study to evaluate reliability of LASCA to measure peripheral blood perfusion in scleroderma patients. Autoimmunity Reviews. 2018;**17**(8):775-780

Chapter 4

Ankylosing Spondylitis and Other Seronegative Arthritis

Balaji Zacharia and Antony Roy

Abstract

Spondyloarthropathies are a group of disorders having some common features. They are characterised by inflammation of the attachment of tendons known as enthesitis. They are common in males. There is a familial occurrence. There is an association with HLA-B 27. Rheumatoid factor will be negative. Axial skeleton involvement in the form of sacroiliitis or spondylitis is common. The common conditions include ankylosing spondylitis, Reiter's disease, psoriatic arthritis, enteropathic arthritis and reactive arthritis. In this chapter we are going to describe the clinical features, evaluation and management of common spondyloarthropathies.

Keywords: spondyloarthropathies, ankylosing spondylitis, enteropathic arthritis, reactive arthritis, psoriatic arthritis

1. Introduction

Spondyloarthropathies are a group of disorders having common clinical features and are characterised by inflammation of the attachment of tendons known as enthesitis. They are common in males and show familial inheritance patterns. The HLA-B 27 allele is frequently associated with these disorders. A rheumatoid factor assay will be negative (seronegative spondyloarthropathy). Axial skeleton involvement in the form of sacroiliitis or spondylitis is common. The common conditions include ankylosing spondylitis, Reiter's disease, psoriatic arthritis, enteropathic arthritis and reactive arthritis [1, 2]. In this chapter we describe the classification, clinical features, evaluation and management of common spondyloarthropathies.

2. Classification

A broad clinical classification of spondyloarthropathies into those having a primary axial involvement, those with a predominant peripheral involvement, and those with a hybrid form of affliction, although eases clinical practise, is difficult to reproduce with uniformity. The current favourite diagnostic criteria, The modified New York criteria for AS is heavily dependent on axial spine affliction and recognises advanced structural damage thus reducing the importance of early extra spinal manifestations, serological evidence and genetic predisposition. There is no emphasis on detection of early radiological manifestations by more informative imaging techniques like magnetic resonance scanning. Inflammatory back pain, the leading clinical symptom of spinal and sacroiliac affliction has been defined by many criteria although its diagnostic significance has not been completely understood and the sensitivity and specificity offered by it is low. It is efficient in diagnosing definite cases although a classification of disease based on it leaves much confusion. The Assessment of SpondyloArthritis International Society axial spondyloarthritis criteria (axSpA) allows for earlier detection of disease thus facilitating earlier disease modification and is more comparable across studies. The focus of treatment in spondyloarthropathies has shifted on to earlier diagnosis and treatment. Magnetic resonance imaging and specific serological tests such as the HLA-B 27 form an essential component of this strategy. In 2011 the ASAS described the peripheral spondyloarthritis criteria specially aimed at the cohort of patients with no or non-specific back pain but with predominant peripheral manifestations [3–5].

3. Ankylosing spondylitis (AS)

This is the prototype disease among spondyloarthropathies. It is also known as Marie-Strumpell disease or Von Bechterew disease. The exact aetiology is unknown. It mainly involves spine and major joints like hip and knee. Sacroiliitis is one of the cardinal features of this disease. It usually affects males in the second or third decade of life. The male to female ratio is 3:1.

There is a striking correlation between AS and HLA-B27 antigen. The disease occurs more frequently in Caucasians where HLA-B27 prevalence is higher as compared to African Americans or Africans of unmixed ancestry. About 1–2% of adults inheriting HLA-B2 antigen have ankylosing spondylitis. In families of patients with AS there is 10–20% prevalence of this antigen. There is no direct causative relationship between HLA-B27 antigen and AS. There is a strong association between AS and inflammatory bowel diseases like ulcerative colitis and Crohn's disease. Both genetic and environmental factors play a role in the pathogenesis of ankylosing spondylitis [6].

3.1 Pathology and pathogenesis

Sacroiliac inflammation is the earliest feature of AS with inflammatory granulation tissue eroding the sacroiliac joint. The inner and thinner iliac cartilage is eroded before the thicker outer sacral sided cartilage. This leads to fibrocartilage tissue replacing the joint space followed by bony ankylosis of sacroiliac joints. There is diffuse osteoporosis of the vertebrae. The inflammation stars at the junction of the intervertebral disc and body. Inflammation and erosion proceeds at the bone disc interface and new bone formation occurs from the edges of the annulus fibrosus known as syndesmophytes. They grow vertically upwards and bridge the adjacent vertebrae producing bamboo spine appearance in radiograph. Early on, inflammation at the bone disc interface produces corner shining sign and later erosion produces squaring of vertebrae. Arthritis of apophyseal joint leads to erosion and later ankylosis of the same. Inflammation and erosion at the sites of attachment of ligaments and tendons are common. Enthesitis followed by calcification is common in the axial skeleton. Unlike in rheumatoid arthritis destruction of central cartilage due to granulation and pannus in peripheral joints can occur in AS. There can be synovitis in peripheral joints.

Extra articular involvement like recurrent uveitis, aortic regurgitation, inflammatory lesions of colon and ileocecal valve and IgA nephropathy are seen in some cases [6, 7].

The exact mechanism of pathogenesis is unknown. It is thought that the destruction is mediated through immunological mechanisms. The elevated levels of inflammatory reactants, Ig A levels in serum and histology suggest inflammation in AS. The exact environmental trigger is not yet identified although elevated levels of antibodies to *Klebsiella pneumoniae* are seen in AS patients. There is no causative association between ankylosing spondylitis and HLA-B27 [8, 9].

3.2 Clinical features

The disease is common in males and in the second and third decade of life. The common presentation in majority of patients is dull aching low back pain which is progressive. There is morning stiffness lasting for few hours and decreased by activity. Pain increasing with rest and improving with exercise is a characteristic feature. Nocturnal exacerbation of pain awakening the patients making them move around is also common. Exacerbations and remissions of symptoms are also common. The enthesitis produces pain in the costochondral junction, greater tuberosity, tibial tuberosity and spinous processes. In some patients the presenting symptom is intractable plantar fasciitis. Neck pain and involvement of cervical spine is late. Sometimes, patients present with features of arthritis in hip or shoulder. Peripheral asymmetrical joint arthritis is rarely seen. Constitutional symptoms like fever, anorexia, weight loss and night sweats can occur rarely.

The common extra articular involvement is ophthalmic. It is usually uni-ocular uveitis. Occasionally it precedes low back symptoms. Red eye, pain, photophobia and increased lacrimation are common. Aortic regurgitation is seen in some patients and can lead to congestive cardiac failure. AS may be associated with inflammatory bowel disease in many patients [8–10].

Tenderness can be elicited over sacroiliac joints, spinous process and areas of enthesitis. The most common feature is loss of mobility of the spine. It is partially due to bony ankylosis and partially due to paraspinal muscle spasms. Forward flexion, lateral rotation and extension of spine are limited. There is loss of lumbar lordosis, increased thoracic kyphosis, flexion deformity of cervical spine flexion deformity of knee. Later this leads to stooping forward posture. This can be demonstrated by occipital wall test. The decreased excursion of lumbar spine movement can be demonstrated by using modified Schober's test. Costovertebral joint involvement can be detected by decreased chest expansion. Sacroiliitis is characterised by local tenderness. Sacroiliac stress test like FABER test, pump handle test can be done though not specific. There can be features of arthritis with ankylosis of hip joints and shoulder. Peripheral joints involvement needs to be evaluated in all cases [8–10].

Earlier onset of disease signals a poor prognosis. They will have severe arthritis of hip. Women have lesser involvement of axial skeleton, mostly isolated involvement of cervical spine and peripheral joints. Due to spinal osteoporosis there can be fractures of spine even with minor trauma. It is common in cervical spine leading to quadriple gia. This is one of the cause of death in AS. There are reports of pulmonary fibrosis, cardiac conduction defects and chronic prostatitis in long standing AS [10, 11].

Restrictive lung disease due to bilateral pulmonary fibrosis can occur. Superadded aspergillosis may mimic tuberculosis. Insertional tendinitis of costosternal and costovertebral muscles leads to pleuritis. Chest expansion is compromised due to fusion of costovertebral joints. There is a threefold increase in risk of death due to respiratory causes in AS patients than in normal people [10, 11].

3.3 Investigations

There is no diagnostic investigation for AS. In the active stage of disease ESR and serum CRP levels are elevated. In severe disease serum alkaline phosphatase will be elevated. Occasionally normocytic normochromic anaemia is associated. There is an elevated IgA level in most cases. HLA-B27 will be elevated. Synovial fluid examination is usually inconclusive. Rheumatoid factor and antinuclear antibodies will be uniformly absent. Pulmonary function tests show reduced vital capacity and increased residual capacity.

Radiograph of the sacroiliac joints shows bilateral involvement. The initial stage is characterised by blurring of the subchondral bone followed by erosion and sclerosis. Progressive erosion produces pseudo widening of the joints. Later progressive bony ankylosis of bilateral sacroiliac joints is seen. These changes are detected by computerised tomography and MRI at an earlier stage than plain radiograph [12].

In the spine there is diffuse osteoporosis. The initial stages show reactive osteitis at the corners of vertebrae producing corner shining sign on lateral view. Later erosion of the corner area produces squaring of the vertebrae. Syndesmophytes growing vertically from the margins of intervertebral disc bridge the adjacent vertebrae and lead to the typical bamboo spine appearance. Lumbar lordosis is lost and dorsal kyphosis is exaggerated.

Articular erosion in the hip leads to features of arthritis and sometimes protrusio acetabuli, later progressing to bony ankylosis. Even though majority of patients have some functional impairment they can lead a fairly normal life [12, 13].

3.4 Diagnosis and differential diagnosis

The most common presenting symptom of AS is inflammatory back pain characterised by pain low back of more than 3 months duration, pain aggregated with inactivity and relieved with activity, presence of morning stiffness and insidious onset in younger patients below the age of 40. But it will be difficult to diagnose AS early before the development of sacroiliitis of spinal deformities. It has been shown that people positive for HLA-B27 developing sacroiliitis at a later date. Because of these difficulties a criteria was developed for the diagnosis of AS. The modified New York criteria consist of (1) history of inflammatory back pain, (2) reduced range of movement of lumbar spine both in frontal and sagittal planes, (3) reduced chest expansion, (4) radiographic evidence of sacroiliitis. The criteria suggest that the presence of radiographic sacroiliitis with any other criteria can make a diagnosis of ankylosing spondylitis.

There are a few conditions which can mimic AS. Diffuse idiopathic skeletal hyperostosis (DISH) is one differential diagnosis but this seen in elderly usually calcification is unilateral on the right side, intervertebral spaces are maintained. Radiogram shows ossified anterior spinal ligament as flowing wax. Fluorosis is another disease but this is usually endemic to certain areas and calcification of sacroiliac and sacrotuberous and other ligamentous calcifications are characteristics. Ochronosis and hemochromatosis can produce intervertebral disc calcification but can be differentiated from AS by other features [14, 15].

3.5 Treatment

There is no medical cure for ankylosing spondylitis. Treatment aims to maintain a functional posture and preserve joint mobility. Exercise can improve and preserve mobility. Swimming and yoga are also helpful. In the active stages NSAIDs especially indomethacin is very useful. Intra-lesional and intra-articular glucocorticoid injections are useful for symptomatic relief of enthesitis or peripheral joint arthritis. Guided glucocorticoid injections are also useful for the relief of sacroiliitis. Sulphasalazine is useful for the long term control of peripheral joint arthritis. Peripheral joint symptoms can also be controlled using methotrexate.

The most common surgical treatment is for hip arthritis. Total hip replacements can improve the pain and joint stiffness. Usually hip involvement produces flexion deformity which leads to flexion of knee. Total hip replacement can improve the gait and posture of patients [14, 15].

A fixed kyphotic deformity at the cervicothoracic junction can lead to chin on chest deformity. This is a rare and disabling condition. A posterior cervicothoracic extension osteotomy can be done for this deformity. It helps in restoration of head and neck posture, relieves pain and improves function. Severe kyphotic deformity of dorsal spine can produce pain and inability to stand straight. This can be managed by an extension osteotomy like Watson Jones osteotomy [16–18].

Mydriatics and local glucocorticoid administration are indicated for iritis. Aortic valve replacement may be needed for aortic valve insufficiency and pacemaker for conduction defects [18].

4. Other spondyloarthropathies

4.1 Reactive arthritis or Reiter's syndrome

It is an acute nonpurulent arthritis occurring following an episode of enteric or urogenital infection in HLA-B27 positive people. Formerly the classical triad of urethritis, arthritis and conjunctivitis was known as Reiter's syndrome. Although Reiter's syndrome is one among the reactive arthritis this term is not used currently. All spondyloarthropathies occurring following urogenital or enteric infections are termed reactive arthritis even if all classical features of Reiter's syndrome are not present. Shigella, Salmonella, Yersinia and Campylobacter are the common organisms that cause enteric infection associated with reactive arthritis. Chlamydia trachomatis is the commonest urogenital infection leading to reactive arthritis. When reactive arthritis occur following a sexually transmitted urogenital infection it is termed as Sexually transmitted associated reactive arthritis (SARS), and when occur following gut related infections called Gut associated reactive arthritis (GARS). There is no gender predilection and occurrence is equal in males and females. Although it can occur at any age, commonly affected are individuals of the age group of 20 to 40 years. Similar to ankylosing spondylitis, there is a close association between HLA-B27 and reactive arthritis [19].

Pathology is similar to other inflammatory arthritis. Enthesitis is also common. Keratoderma blenorrhagica is a skin condition associated with reactive arthritis especially with urogenital infections. The exact triggering mechanism for the pathogenesis of reactive arthritis is unknown. There are reports of acute nonpurulent arthritis associated with bacterial, viral and even parasitic infections. Like in ankylosing spondylitis it is mediated through immunological mechanisms. There is persistence of organism in the inflamed synovium for prolonged duration although not demonstrated in blood. The role of HLA-B27 also remains unclear.

4.2 Clinical features

The clinical features can range from mild mono articular involvement to asymmetrical poly articular arthritis. Most patients will give a history of antecedent infection either in the GI tract or urogenital region. Sometimes, there is a history of sexual promiscuity. In males, urethritis or prostatitis and in females cervicitis or salpingitis may be present though asymptomatic. Unlike ankylosing spondylitis, constitutional symptoms like fatigue, malaise, fever are common in reactive arthritis. The arthritis typically involves the lower limb joints. Knee, ankle, subtalar, metatarsophalangeal joints and inter-phalangeal joints are commonly involved. There is asymmetrical involvement and usually migrates from one joint to another over a period. Wrist and fingers can also be involved. Painfull joints with tense effusion are common especially in large joints like knee. Dactylitis with sausage digits can occur in single or multiple fingers. Enthesitis producing symptoms of insertional tendo achilles tendinitis and plantar fasciitis can be seen. Low back pain due to sacroiliitis, enthesitis is also seen [20].

Extra articular lesions like conjunctivitis and severe uveitis can cause blindness in certain patients with reactive arthritis. Vesicular and hyperkeratotic lesions seen in hand and foot are called Keratoderma blenorrhagica. Circinate balanitis of glans penis is also described. Like in ankylosing spondylitis aortic regurgitation, cardiac conduction defects and pulmonary involvement can rarely occur [21].

4.3 Investigations

In the acute phase there will be elevated ESR and CRP. Synovial fluid analysis is inconclusive. Occasionally there is a marked elevation of antibodies to salmonella, chlamydia and yersinia indicating recent infections with these organisms.

Radiograph will be normal in early cases. Later on, peri-articular osteoporosis develops in chronic cases followed by juxtaarticular erosions and loss of joint space. New bone formation due to periostitis can occur. Spur formation at the attachments of tendons are also seen. Sacroiliitis and spondylitis occur very late and are uncommon. Sacroiliitis is unilateral and asymmetrical. Unlike in ankylosing spondylitis the spondylitis may not show an ascending pattern and it can involve any level. The syndesmophytes may be coarse and nonmarginal arising from the middle of vertebrae. Spinal fusion is very rare [21, 22].

4.4 Diagnosis and differential diagnosis

Diagnosis is based on clinical examination as there is no confirmatory laboratory test available. A careful history of recent infection in the gut and urogenital tract is to be elicited. Careful examination of genitalia, eye, skin, nail and mucous membranes must be done. In doubtful cases HLA-B27 testing can be done [23].

The most common differential diagnosis is gonococcal arthritis. But it involves both lower and upper limbs equally. Low back pain is not seen in gonococcal arthritis. Characteristic vesicular skin lesions are common. Culturing gonococci from blood, skin lesion or synovium establishes the diagnosis. Psoriatic arthritis is another differential diagnosis [24].

Undifferentiated spondyloarthropathies can present like reactive arthritis. They may present with isolated arthritis involving knee, ankle or dactylitis or enthesitis like plantar fasciitis and insertional tendo achilles tendinitis. They may not meet the diagnostic characteristic of other classical spondyloarthropathies. Approximately half of patients with undifferentiated spondyloarthropathies are HLA-B27 positive [23, 24].

4.5 Treatment

Most patients with reactive arthritis respond well to NSAIDS for symptomatic relief. Indomethacin 75–150 mg in divided doses is the initial treatment of choice. Sulphasalazine up to 3 g/day may be helpful especially patients not responding to NSAIDS. Immunosuppressive agents such as azathioprine 1–2 mg/kg per day and methotrexate 7.5–15 mg per week are useful. Tendinitis and enthesitis can be treated with intra lesional glucocorticoid injections. Uveitis may require aggressive treatment with glucocorticoid to prevent blindness [21, 23].

5. Psoriatic arthritis

Since the association between HLA-B27 and psoriatic spondylitis (60%) is less when compared to AS (94%) it is included in spondyloarthropathies. About 2% of individuals having psoriasis develop arthritis. Peripheral arthritis is common than axial disease. In majority of patients skin lesions predate arthritis. But in one fourth of cases the skin lesions appear simultaneously or arthritis predate skin lesions. In such cases a there may be a family history of psoriasis. Nail changes like ridging, pitting and onycholysis are common in psoriatic arthritis. Though psoriatic distal inter-phalangeal joint arthritis is common in males incidence is similar in both sexes. There are many forms of psoriatic arthritis [25].

1. Oligoarticular disease (70%): it is the most common type of psoriatic arthritis. Asymmetrical arthritis involving the lower limb joints is common. It can involve small joints of fingers. Both distal and proximal inter-phalangeal joints are involved- sausage fingers. Lack of distal inter-phalangeal joint involvement helps to differentiate it from rheumatoid arthritis. Nail changes are frequent in fingers having distal inter-phalangeal involvement.

2. Symmetrical polyarthritis (15%): it may be indistinguishable from rheumatoid arthritis. But presence of rheumatoid nodules and distal inter-phalangeal joint involvement and positive rheumatoid factor helps to distinguish it from rheumatoid arthritis.

3. Arthritis mutilans (5–10%): it is a severe destructive asymmetrical arthritis. It is usually seen in severe form of psoriasis. It is associated with sacroiliitis and spondylitis.

4. Psoriatic spondylitis (25%): it is strongly associated with HLA-B27 (60%). Majority of cases are asymptomatic. Asymmetrical sacroiliitis is common. Spondylitis without sacroiliitis producing florid syndesmophyte formation is common in psoriasis.

Features like distal inter-phalangeal joint involvement, absent peri articular osteoporosis, periostitis, ankylosis, pencil in cup deformities of DIP joints and axial skeleton involvement in radiograph help to differentiate it from rheumatoid arthritis. Sometimes, concomitant gouty arthritis can be seen even in premenopausal women due to high skin cell turnover [26, 27].

5.1 Treatment

Majority of cases are oligoarticular and mild and have good prognosis. NSAIDS are the mainstay of symptomatic treatment. Intra-articular glucocorticoid injections are helpful in oligoarticular disease. Methotrexate and azathioprine are useful for long term control of both skin and arthritic lesions. Antimalarial and systemic steroids must be avoided for the fear of exacerbation of skin lesions [28].

6. Enteropathic arthritis

Seronegative spondyloarthropathies can occur in association with inflammatory bowel disorders (IBD). They are twice commonly associated with Crohn's disease than ulcerative colitis. Two forms of peripheral arthritis are described.

Type 1: it is strongly associated with extra intestinal manifestations of IBD. It is usually pauciarticular and is seen during relapses of IBD. It is acute and self-limiting.

Type 2: more than five joints are involved. It runs a chronic course lasting for years independent of the IBD. Uveitis can occur but other extra intestinal manifestations are rare.

Extra articular manifestations like erythema nodosum, pyoderma gangrenosum, aphthous stomatitis can occur. Exact pathogenesis of enteropathic arthritis is not known. Increased gut permeability leading to entry of bacilli from gut into general circulation and immune mediated mechanism is one proposed theory [29, 30].

6.1 Treatment

There will be intolerance to NSAIDS due to gastrointestinal involvement. Hence simple analgesics are used. Intra-articular glucocorticoid injections are useful. Sulfasalazine is useful for the control of both arthritis and gut disease. Systemic corticosteroids, methotrexate and azathioprine are also used [30, 31].

6.2 Biological DMARDs in spondyloarthropathies

Treatment with biological agents is used in patients who fail to respond to NSAIDs. It should be started at an early stage to prevent progression. Tumour necrosis factor alpha inhibitors are the commonest drugs used. They prevent cartilage damage in peripheral joints than in axial joints. These drugs reduce the radiographic progression of disease in AS when administered early. Highest response to these drugs occurred in psoriatic arthritis patients with elevated CRP levels. Due to fear of reactivation it is always better to screen for the presence of latent tuberculosis or hepatic viral diseases [30]. In addition to biological agents the ASAS recommends a single local corticosteroid injection in cases of peripheral spondyloarthritis.

7. Tumour necrosis factor alpha inhibitors

Etanercept, infliximab, adalimumab, golimumab, certolizumab are the common TNF alpha inhibitors used. Infliximab is used intravenously and the others are administered subcutaneously. They are effective for spondyloarthropathies and psoriatic arthritis which are not controlled by NSAIDS and traditional DMARDS. Certolizumab, a recent drug is effective in reducing the symptoms and axial involvement in AS. Infliximab, adalimumab, golimumab are used in IBD to treat both bowel and joint diseases. Etanercept is useful in controlling axial skeleton involvement but its effect on enteric disease is limited. Infliximab and adalimumab used in AS have shown to decrease the rate of recurrences. Golimumab is found to be effective in refractory uveitis associated with spondyloarthropathies. TNF-alpha inhibitors like infliximab, adalimumab, golimumab, and etanercept are very efficient in treating the skin and nail lesions in psoriasis though exacerbations of lesions can occur rarely with TNF alpha inhibitors. TNF alpha inhibitors decrease cardiovascular manifestations. In AS, the overall treatment with biological DMARDS shows only partial remission or low disease activity [32–34].

Interleukin-6 receptor inhibitors like Tocilizumab and Sarilumab are found to be not effective in the treatment of spondyloarthropathies by various trials. A shotterm study involving 30 patients with AS treated using Secukinumab showed its clinical efficacy but need to be confirmed by long term RCTS. Ustekinumab, a fully human monoclonal antibody against a common subunit of lL12 and IL 23, is well tolerated and found to be effective in AS and psoriatic arthritis [35].

8. Current consensus and the way forward

The 2016 update on Assessment of SpondyloArthritis international Society (ASAS)-European league against rheumatism (EULAR) recommendations provide guidance on the management of patients with axial spondyloarthritis. A total of five broad principles of management and treatment recommendations have been put forward. They are precise guidelines to treat patients with axial spondyloarthropathies broadly incorporating therapeutic and diagnostic concerns [36].

9. Conclusion

Spondyloarthropathies are a group of conditions having some common overlapping clinical features. They are common in HLA-B27 antigen positive individuals. There is no conclusive investigation for these conditions hence differentiation is difficult at least in the early stages. For most of the cases only symptomatic treatments are available. Further research is needed for early detection and accurate treatment of these conditions.

Author details

Balaji Zacharia* and Antony Roy
Department of Orthopaedics, Government Medical College, Kozhikode, Kerala, India

*Address all correspondence to: balaji.zacharia@gmail.com

References

[1] Howe HS et al. Seronegative spondyloarthropathy—Studies from the Asia Pacific region. Annals of the Academy of Medicine (Singapore). 2007;**36**(2):135-141

[2] Shankarkumar U, Devraj JP, Ghosh K, Mohanty D. Seronegative spondarthritis and human leucocyte antigen association. British Journal of Biomedical Science. 2002;**59**(1):38-41

[3] van Tubergen A, Weber U. Diagnosis and classification in spondyloarthritis: Identifying a chameleon. Nature Reviews Rheumatology. 2012;**8**(5): 253-261. DOI: 10.1038/nrrheum.2012.33

[4] Sieper J. Developments in therapies for spondyloarthritis. Nature Reviews Rheumatology. 2012;**8**(5):280-287. DOI: 10.1038/nrrheum.2012.40

[5] Akgul O, Ozgocmen S. Classification criteria for spondyloarthropathies. World Journal of Orthopedics. 2011;**2**(12):107-115

[6] Haroon N. Ankylosis in ankylosing spondylitis: Current concepts. Clinical Rheumatology. 2015;**34**(6):1003-1007. DOI: 10.1007/s10067-015-2956-4

[7] de Koning A, Schoones JW, van der Heijde D, van Gaalen FA. Pathophysiology of axial spondyloarthritis: Consensus and controversies. European Journal of Clinical Investigation. 2018;**48**(5):e12913. DOI: 10.1111/eci.12913

[8] Shamji MF, Bafaquh M, Tsai E. The pathogenesis of ankylosing spondylitis. Neurosurgical Focus. 2008;**24**(1):E3. DOI: 10.3171/FOC/2008/24/1/E3

[9] Rashid T, Ebringer A, Wilson C. The link between klebsiella and ankylosing spondylitis in worldwide geographical locations. Current Rheumatology Reviews. 2016;**12**(3):223-231

[10] Smith JA. Update on ankylosing spondylitis: Current concepts in pathogenesis. Current Allergy and Asthma Reports. 2015;**15**(1):489. DOI: 10.1007/s11882-014-0489-6

[11] Sieper J, Braun J, Rudwaleit M, Boonen A, Zink A. Ankylosing spondylitis: An overview. Annals of the Rheumatic Diseases. 2002;**61**(Suppl 3): iii8-iii18

[12] Kim Y, Oh HC, Park JW, et al. Diagnosis and treatment of inflammatory joint disease. Hip and Pelvis. 2017;**29**(4):211-222. DOI: 10.5371/hp.2017.29.4.211

[13] Poddubnyy D, Sieper J. Similarities and differences between nonradiographic and radiographic axial spondyloarthritis: A clinical, epidemiological and therapeutic assessment. Current Opinion in Rheumatology. 2014;**26**(4):377-383. DOI: 10.1097/BOR.0000000000000071

[14] Taurog JD, Chhabra A, Colbert RA. Ankylosing spondylitis and axial spondyloarthritis. The New England Journal of Medicine. 2016;**374**(26):2563-2574. DOI: 10.1056/NEJMra1406182

[15] Braun J, Sieper J. Ankylosing spondylitis. Lancet. 2007;**369**(9570):1379-1390

[16] Liu H, Yang C, Zheng Z, Ding W, Wang J, Wang H, et al. Comparison of Smith-Petersen osteotomy and pedicle subtraction osteotomy for the correction of thoracolumbar kyphotic deformity in ankylosing spondylitis: A systematic review and meta-analysis. Spine (Phila., PA, 1976). 2015;**40**(8):570-579. DOI: 10.1097/BRS.0000000000000815

[17] Moon KH, Kim YT. Medical treatment of ankylosing spondylitis. Hip and Pelvis. 2014;**26**(3):129-135. DOI: 10.5371/hp.2014.26.3.129

[18] Ho HH, Chen JY. Ankylosing spondylitis: Chinese perspective, clinical phenotypes, and associated extra-articular systemic features. Current Rheumatology Reports. 2013;**15**(8):344. DOI: 10.1007/s11926-013-0344-0

[19] Kvien TK, Glennås A, Melby K, Granfors K, Andrup O, Karstensen B, et al. Reactive arthritis: Incidence, triggering agents and clinical presentation. The Journal of Rheumatology. 1994 Jan;**21**(1):115-122

[20] Schmitt SK. Reactive arthritis. Infectious Disease Clinics of North America. 2017;**31**(2):265-277. DOI: 10.1016/j.idc.2017.01.002

[21] Carter JD, Hudson AP. Reactive arthritis: Clinical aspects and medical management. Rheumatic Diseases Clinics of North America. 2009;**35**(1):21-44. DOI: 10.1016/j.rdc.2009.03.010

[22] Townes JM. Reactive arthritis after enteric infections in the United States: The problem of definition. Clinical Infectious Diseases. 2010;**50**(2):247-254. DOI: 10.1086/649540

[23] Carter JD. Bacterial agents in spondyloarthritis: A destiny from diversity? Best Practice and Research: Clinical Rheumatology. 2010;**24**(5):701-714. DOI: 10.1016/j.berh.2010.05.002

[24] Selmi C, Gershwin ME. Diagnosis and classification of reactive arthritis. Autoimmunity Reviews. 2014;**13**(4-5):546-549. DOI: 10.1016/j.autrev.2014.01.005

[25] Ruderman EM. Evaluation and management of psoriatic arthritis: The role of biologic therapy. Journal of the American Academy of Dermatology. 2003;**49**(2 Suppl):S125-S132

[26] Sharma A, Dogra S. Management of psoriatic arthritis. Indian Journal of Dermatology, Venereology and Leprology. 2010;**76**(6):645-651. DOI: 10.4103/0378-6323.72457

[27] Balakrishnan C, Madnani N. Diagnosis and management of psoriatic arthritis. Indian Journal of Dermatology, Venereology and Leprology. 2013;**79**(Suppl 7):S18-S24. DOI: 10.4103/0378-6323.115507

[28] Pipitone N, Kingsley GH, Manzo A, Scott DL, Pitzalis C. Current concepts and new developments in the treatment of psoriatic arthritis. Rheumatology (Oxford, England). 2003;**42**(10): 1138-1148. [Epub Jun 16, 2003]

[29] Peluso R, Di Minno MND, Iervolino S, et al. Enteropathic spondyloarthritis: From diagnosis to treatment. Clinical and Developmental Immunology. 2013;**2013**:631408. DOI: 10.1155/2013/631408

[30] Peluso R, Manguso F, Vitiello M, Iervolino S, Di Minno MND. Management of arthropathy in inflammatory bowel diseases. Therapeutic Advances in Chronic Disease. 2015;**6**(2):65-77. DOI: 10.1177/2040622314563929

[31] Speca S, Dubuquoy L. Chronic bowel inflammation and inflammatory joint disease: Pathophysiology. Joint, Bone, Spine. 2017;**84**(4):417-420. DOI: 10.1016/j.jbspin.2016.12.016. [Epub Jan 3, 2017]

[32] Braun J, Kiltz U, Heldmann F, Baraliakos X. Emerging drugs for the treatment of axial and peripheral spondyloarthritis. Expert Opinion on Emerging Drugs. 2015;**20**(1):1-14. DOI: 10.1517/14728214.2015.993378

[33] Papagoras C, Voulgari PV, Drosos AA. Golimumab, the newest TNF-α blocker, comes of age. Clinical and Experimental Rheumatology. 2015;**33**(4):570-577

[34] Toussirot E. New treatment options and emerging drugs for axial

spondyloarthritis: Biological and targeted synthetic agents. Expert Opinion on Pharmacotherapy. 2017;**18**(3):275-282. DOI: 10.1080/14656566.2017.1284793

[35] Cauli A, Piga M, Lubrano E, Marchesoni A, Floris A, Mathieu A. New approaches in tumour necrosis factor antagonism for the treatment of psoriatic arthritis: Certolizumab pegol. The Journal of Rheumatology. 2015;**93**:70-72. DOI: 10.3899/jrheum.150641

[36] van der Heijde D, Ramiro S, Landewé R, et al. Update of the ASAS-EULAR management recommendations for axial spondyloarthritis. Annals of the Rheumatic Diseases. 2017;**76**:978-991

Chapter 5

Physical Exercise Improves Quality of Life in Patients with Connective Tissue Disease

Ricardo Munir Nahas, Vivianne Horsti Dos Santos and Silvio Lopes Alabarse

Abstract

Connective tissue diseases (CTDs) affect the parts of the body that connect the structures of the body components together. As the conditions involve inflammatory responses in the joints, tendons, ligaments, skin, cornea, cartilage, bones, muscles and blood vessels, which cause symptoms of rheumatism, the CTDs can also be referred to as rheumatic diseases. The symptoms include pain, swelling, redness, warmth in a joint or affected area and functional loss of motion. The medical domain for these types of disorders is called rheumatology. Among various conditions fell under the broad heading of rheumatism, the common rheumatic disorders that here we take care of are rheumatoid arthritis (RA), systemic lupus erythematosus (SLE), scleroderma (S), systemic sclerosis (SS), polymyositis/dermatomyositis (PM/DM), spondyloarthropathies (SA) (ankylosing spondylitis (AS) and psoriatic arthritis (PsA)), juvenile idiopathic arthritis (JIA), polymyalgia rheumatica (PMR), Sjogren's syndrome, osteoarthritis, etc. When the diagnosis of CTDs is made by the rheumatologists, they oversee a treatment plan for the patients, which may include not only medications but also physical exercises. In this chapter, we will describe how the physical exercise contributes to the patients who suffered from CTDs. Furthermore, we intend to explain what type of exercise should be performed as well as its intensity, duration frequency and the benefits of those exercises to the health of those patients.

Keywords: connective tissue disease, exercise, intensity, lifestyle, prior participation

1. Introduction

Therapeutic with regular controlled exercise has been widely employed in a range of disease treatments that involves a broad range of causes and various effects on the human body. Studies show that physical activity and regular exercise in association with specific medications provide greater longevity and improve the quality in the treatment and prevention of disease when compared to groups that do not integrate exercise into their daily lifestyle. The case of CTD is no distinct. The aggressive effects of autoimmune and degenerative diseases on the connective tissue of the locomotive apparatus directly reflect on patients' ability to perform physical exercise. The physical capacity of these patients is lower when compared to sedentary individuals who do not have any type of disease. This is due to the functional limitations caused by the deformities, fixed or not, and mainly by the pain that the movements impose on the patients. Patients with their connective tissue, affected by degenerative or autoimmune diseases, are subject to periods of acute crisis that make simple movements painful and more elaborate movements impossible. Consequently, it makes the physical activity practice a challenge [1–3].

Another important aspect to be highlighted is fatigue in these patients. This group tires more quickly, especially when they are compared to sedentary individuals without systemic diseases or other physical limitations. The more sedentary the patients with connective tissue diseases are, the less they can tolerate effort, and sooner they get fatigued. It is important to emphasize that sometimes these diseases have a differential diagnosis for pain syndromes observed in elite competitive athletes. In other words, patients are mistakenly diagnosed as having sports injuries. This error can lead to a higher period away from the practice of sport since initial treatment is not compatible with the underlying and neglected disease [2, 3].

In this sense, this chapter aims to show not only the benefits that regular exercise can have for this group of patients in terms of connective tissue but also what type of exercise should be performed and at what intensity, duration and weekly frequency. It also encourages the assisting physician to prescribe regular physical activities, which complements treating diseases of the connective tissue, being a powerful ally of essential pharmaceutical treatment. Controlled physical activity minimizes the effects of these diseases in acute crises as well as in terms of controlling the signs and symptoms involved in the chronic progression of the disease. Exercise is also a preventive method to delay the onset of connective tissue degeneration as well as to interspace acute crises, becoming less frequent [3, 4].

2. Specific assessment prior to participation

A medical evaluation to identify limitations and correct deformities (whether fixed or not) is fundamental and should be performed by the assisting physician, who will prescribe the restrictions to the practice of physical activity and exercises. This step is crucial to avoid training mistakes and further progress of diseases. Once the underlying disease (autoimmune or degenerative) is determined, questions that provide information about the level of physical activity in the patient's daily life are important in order to understand how sedentary he or she is as well as the number of steps the patient takes each day. During this initial contact, the patient should state which of the joint (or joints) is (are) more affected and more painful and whether the pain is related to work, leisure activities or both. In addition, notes of the approximate interval between acute disease crises will serve as feedback for treatment involving exercise. With exercises, these crises will tend to become farther apart, and this type of information is important for patients to adhere to treatment [5].

Identifying the story of sports and exercises practised so far will help to prescribe the best type of motion to the patient. The memory of movement will make the difference in selecting the future route to be followed. For instance, prescribing aquatic exercises is an alternative for those patients, who have never been in a pool or who are likely to abandon treatment.

During the physical examination, the physician might have an accurate idea of how much balance and coordination the patient has even its standing and sitting posture. This can be confirmed by the axial skeleton, potential lateral and anteroposterior deviations of the spinal column, anterior and posterior scales of the scapula and pelvic ring beyond the alignment of the arms and legs, all resulting from mechanical causes (agonist and antagonist muscle imbalances). The range of motion in affected and unaffected joints should be recorded, mainly in the lower limbs. Whether it is possible, deformities must be treated prior to or alongside therapy, in order to address pain or functional limitations [5]. The arm, forearm, thigh and leg circumference measures should be taken, and an evaluation of the secondary stability that muscular strength can offer to the joints will be useful as a parameter to measure changes in physical capacity.

Observing the gait of patients during short displacement and their ability to sit down and stand up contributes to a better understanding of essential physical needs in the routine life of patients. In relation to the subsidiary exams, which are directly relevant to an efficient orientation of the best activity to be performed, we highlight the treadmill or cycle ergometer test. The maximum effort achieved allows better determination of the heart rate interval for the practice of aerobic exercise that will be prescribed.

Clinically speaking, the evaluation of cardiovascular function in stress tests may also cause cardiac function alterations and diseases that eventually exacerbate during more intense efforts, which had been performed before. The exercise prescription will be more accurate when the values for oxygen consumption, aerobic and anaerobic thresholds and maximum consumption are obtained over the appointment with a physician.

In addition, body composition measurements are very useful for identifying the loss of muscle mass (sarcopenia), which can be expected from diseases that develop chronically. Similarly, body composition is an extremely important examination since it evaluates the quantity of stored body fat (particularly the amount of visceral fat), a measurement of the excess of weight, which directly affects joints in the legs and worsens degenerative conditions [4, 5].

3. What can be expected from the type of exercise for each physical quality developed?

The type of physical activities and exercises practised can be classified according to how the energy is produced by the muscle responsible for this movement. The aerobic energy production system is the main responsible for long-duration work involving strong resistance. The anaerobic system of energy production, on the other hand, is mainly responsible for power, strength and speed, offering short bursts of energy during movement. In general, a combination of both systems of energy production is used to execute various tasks and always depends on the stimulation offered.

Here we will differentiate the types of movement and their application as an adjuvant in treating autoimmune and degenerative diseases of the connective tissue.

3.1 Aerobic resistance

Overall, the physical capacity should receive more attention from physicians and patients because of the increased benefits it provides to the sedentary and sick people, and it should be no different in patients with connective tissue diseases. This factor will require the most attention in any regular physical training programme, especially for younger and older adults. With this physical work, we seek improvement in the endothelial dysfunction caused by atherosclerosis, which is generally more significant in autoimmune diseases and degenerative arthritis than in the sedentary population. Atherosclerosis is also responsible for the increase in blood pressure, insulin intolerance and diabetes type II, and all can be aggravated by obesity, which in turn becomes more accentuated with a sedentary lifestyle [4].

Patients with connective tissue diseases have less physical capacity than sedentary individuals who do not practice regular exercise. The consequently reduced mobility aggravates their capacity to carry out tasks, even the simplest daily routines. The greater sensation of fatigue, common in patients with early onset connective tissue diseases, decreases in trained individuals when compared to the population in general [6].

In addition, the rise in aerobic capacity has also a fundamental role in diminishing the variation in heart rate. This occurs in trained individuals and requires less effort by the cardiovascular system, with lower energy costs in carrying out the same task. The number of mitochondria in cardiac muscle fibers can be up to five times greater than those contained in the skeletal muscle, and training will yield additional benefits for cardiac function.

After determining the maximum oxygen consumption capacity in this population, the start of training can be planned as well as its evolution, which should be slow and progressive. More intense stimuli for expanding energy gains (and greater benefits) should always be offered when the body reaches a state of balance at a new level. Increasing loads also interest patients who wish to participate in sports and competitions. In controlling disease, these loads are sometimes eliminated as soon as the autonomy of movement and disease control is shown to be effective [6].

Alongside the improved physical capacity obtained with regular exercise, the pain, so far, presented in the life of these patients will diminish. Joint swelling and sensitivity in the affected regions also decrease as a result of improved venous return and better peripheral circulation. The direct impact on better quality of life is remarkable. Mood variations that come from improved self-esteem and better quality of sleep (which is more relaxing and restorative) can also be perceived in patients who practice regular exercise. These encourage patients to adhere to exercise and sports [7].

Regarding the intensity of aerobic exercise, the World Health Organization recommends that aerobic training should be performed at moderate intensity, with heart rate oscillating between the aerobic and anaerobic thresholds (roughly represents around 60 and 80% of the aerobic exercise intensity maximal heart rate), which has direct relation to maximal oxygen consumption (VO2max). The physiological objective of this type of training is not only to raise maximum oxygen consumption (VO_{2max}) levels (increasing maximum work capacity) but also to expand the thresholds and consequently promote greater efficiency during the aerobic resistance exercise. Consequently, it will be reflected in the improvement in health as a whole and, in particular, for connective tissue disease in particular. For patients with a low aerobic capacity due to years of inactivity and sedentary lifestyles, who have been affected by disease symptoms, beginning a programme of regular physical activity may seem impossible. These patients often prefer not to leave their homes and become dependent on their relatives or friends, requiring assistance in all activities [8, 9].

These patients must take on the challenges of their day to day as the beginning of their recovery for independence. Simple tasks such as leaving the house on foot to purchase groceries, taking the stairs to the next floor and walking greater distances to access transport (even slowly and even if this means walking to the patient's own car in a parking area) trigger initial effects and can help stimulate the practice of exercise in the near future.

In some cases, patients may require constant monitoring by specialized staff and daily stimuli to maintain minimal levels of activity. Even if this is done remotely, through messages or phone calls, regular exercise should be encouraged; and the patient will feel obliged to carry out the assigned task. Although they may be less frequent, acute crises may occur. At these times, the intensity of training should be reduced. Movements should be adapted temporarily, and equipment may even be changed (replacing running with bicycling, for example) in order to stop the patient from becoming sedentary once again [9].

3.1.1 Equipment for aerobic resistance training

Once the intensity and cardiac frequency range for the patient's training has been determined, the type of resistance should be chosen. In other words, the type of equipment that will be used should be established. Walking and/or running (either outdoors or on the treadmill), cycling on a stationary or traditional bicycle, swimming and rowing are the most frequent methods chosen for aerobic resistance training.

Since the different movements and specificity (which are important in sports) are not the objective of the training, varying the type of movement is interesting because it moves different muscle groups, making exercise less routine. This may occur when swimming is replaced with running, for instance. For some types of exercises, the memory of movement is essential. These exercises require more advanced coordination and balance than others. It is often difficult for an adult to learn to ride a bicycle, even if it is stationary, which makes prescribing this exercise unfeasible. This is even more difficult when swimming is chosen as the exercise [9].

The easiest and most natural exercise for all patients is walking and/or running. The limitations of this mode are excess body weight and the conditions of the cartilage in the leg joints bearing this burden as well as the ability to work the muscle groups in these limbs which may be weakened from disuse. The natural alternative for overweight patients (or even those who are not) and joints that cannot support them is cycling. A stationary bicycle is better because it allows us to efficiently control the speed that will be constant (approximately 30 km/h or 70 revolutions per minute) and a load that is compatible with the desired proportional heart rate and oxygen consumption.

Cycling provides the best gateway to starting a regular aerobic physical activity when there is a need to compensate the reduced muscle resistance in supporting and carrying body weight (and frequently, excessive body weight). The benefits will be felt quickly. Like all equipment, bicycle requires some care in its use. The height of the saddle must be correctly positioned between the perineal region and the ground, avoiding unnecessary stress (particularly on the knees). Handlebars should be correctly positioned with the patient sitting comfortably in the saddle and should allow the rider to gaze towards the horizon. This arrangement will not lead to unwanted stress on lordosis and kyphosis when the line of the axial skeleton is abnormally positioned [10].

If for any reason, the patient cannot cycle, walk or run regularly, walking in the water can be an option. The greater density of water makes the body lighter, while offers resistance to achieve the desired training. The only requirement is to control heart rate and to use floats in order to allow the patient to reproduce the natural movement practised over an entire lifetime. It is always necessary to be careful with fatigue, which appears more quickly in this group of arthritic patients. The lower muscle mass of the arm muscles (in comparison with the legs) yields less efficiency in training for aerobic resistance. This makes this alternative an exception

When incapacitating mechanical alterations make arm exercises the only option, rowing seems to be the best alternative to exercising. This modality requires specific coordination but is easier to perform than swimming, for instance. This can be done traditionally on the water or on equipment that simulates this activity and allows the intensity of the exercise to be controlled. Because it combines leg and arm movements, swimming is a good alternative; nonetheless, specific conditions are required for this to be part of efficient training. Because of the horizontal position of the patient and the fact that water is denser than air, the maximum heart rate achieved in water is lower than in tests performed on the ground. For sedentary patients, you must deduct 13 beats per minute from the values obtained during these tests or from the VO_{2max} determined mathematically [7, 8].

Swimming requires knowledge (movement memory), and this style of exercise may be chosen as a function of biomechanical limitations that may be present in the arms as well as the legs. It may be necessary for the exercise sessions to take place in a location where immediate assistance can be provided and where the staff is trained to work with a population that has limitations imposed by disease in order to prevent accidents. The monitoring of progress during training is more difficult, particularly in terms of exercise intensity. This applies equally to the patient and to those supervising the patient. Remember that this group fatigues earlier than the population in general and that supervision should be attentive and constant.

Because of the adversities involved in the exercises mentioned up to this point, the natural choice is walking or running, since it is more practical and easier to implement and monitor and does not require special or sophisticated equipment. It is universal and can be done indoors or outdoors, and it is the most commonly practised individual sport around the world. It is important to mention that all aerobic work should be done individually. Groups that form around the activity should be social in nature. The intensity of work will always be obtained and applied individually.

Calculations of heart rate, at the beginning of the training (for patients who were sedentary or who had clinical complications interrupt the practice of exercise), should establish a heart rate for oxygen consumption of approximately 50% of maximum capacity (VO_{2max}), which is a lower level than the levels to sedentary people without degenerative diseases. It is explained by the fact that these patients fatigue earlier [9, 10].

In order to maintain the ideal weekly volume of training and considering a lower and more comfortable intensity to the exercises, the session length can be increased, or more sessions can be added per week. The time for each session can be divided and carried out over the space of the same day. As clinical conditions permit and conditioning increases tolerance to fatigue, higher levels of oxygen consumption (higher VO_{2max} percentages) will be offered as a stimulus, always remaining in the moderate activity range between the anaerobic and aerobic thresholds obtained directly or via mathematical calculations. Outdoor exercise makes this activity more playful and should be encouraged, especially when the weather conditions are favorable. Training should begin on soft and flat terrain with few curves. Participants should change direction regularly.

The heart rate controls the pace of intensity during the activity. This may be reflected in a speed that only allows walking during the entire course.

As the patient improves, walking will gradually alternate with small periods of jogging and running, until the patient jogs or runs the entire trajectory. These characteristics make outdoor exercise more individualized. Groups can gather at the beginning and the end of training during warm-up and cool-down activities, but not during the workout. Competitive practices may be indicated for those patients who need individual limits to surpass. It is important that they always be aware of their limitations and tendency towards earlier fatigue [8–10].

3.1.2 Duration and frequency of aerobic exercise

In order to obtain the weekly volume of exercise to be practised by the patient, the intensity of the aerobic resistance training should be added to the time it is performed per session and the number of sessions that will be repeated over the space of a week. It is essential that the pace of each workout be reached gradually and slowly until the desired heart rate is reached (warm-up). At this intensity, start marking time without worrying about the distance traveled. The World Health Organization and the American College of Sports Medicine suggest practising moderate aerobic exercise for an average of 150 minutes per week. These same organizations suggest reducing this time for the week by 50% if the exercise is vigorous. This more intense training should be avoided, especially during periods of connective tissue disease crisis. For more advanced patients, however, this might be an alternative.

The distribution per session must include periods of recovery that integrate the benefits of physical activity and tissue renewal. With this in mind, we suggest dividing the 150 minutes into up to 6 sessions per week and the 75 minutes into up to 5 sessions per week for the determined intensities. For beginners, we suggest training on alternate days and at moderate intensity. We must account for earlier fatigue and muscular hypotrophy, which may require adaptations. Alternating between light and moderate effort can be an interesting option.

If the patient continues to have problems on tolerating exercise, dividing the session into morning and evening activities on the same day can be an interesting alternative (30 minutes broken down into two 15-minute periods, for example). Warm-up and cool-down periods are required for each one of these training periods [10].

3.2 Localized exercises

Muscle loss does not seem to be directly correlated with degenerative and autoimmune diseases, nonetheless, with the progressive inactivity developed over years of disease crisis and its impact on joint function, in addition to disabling pain. To better monitor physical development in patients performing localized exercises and test the efficiency of their training, it is important to quantify the amount of muscle tissue. The results of body composition calculations are often shocking.

Depending on the degree of muscular involvement (when sarcopenia is diagnosed), physical rehabilitation through localized resistance exercises and muscle strength may need to precede the initiation of a broader programme of regular physical activity, such as the aerobic training proposed in the previous item, for example. This step requires the supervision of a professional in the area of rehabilitation.

3.2.1 Localized muscle exercises

Independent work boosts localized muscular strength and endurance while it completes aerobic exercise in an attempt to provide a better quality of life for these patients. The anti-gravitational muscle groups are the focus since they involve large amounts of muscle tissue and are secondary joint stabilizers that keep the body in an orthostatic position. To do so, the gluteal, ischiotibial ("hamstrings"), quadriceps and triceps surae muscles should be assessed and prepared to sustain body weight during essential movement activities, whether these are walking, running, swimming or cycling [11].

Starting the programme with isometric muscle exercises can provide benefits in terms of gains in strength and endurance, with lower overload in the joint affected by connective tissue diseases. As strength and muscle resistance are worked, gains can even be seen in balance and coordination for movement and tasks in everyday life. And as the patient gains autonomy and strength, localized muscular resistance exercises will replace isometric ones.

Regardless of the modality, resistance exercises must be performed in a closed kinetic chain, allowing greater control and coordination of the patient over the movement, which is to be performed. Because of the limitations of the disease itself, each series will contain more repetitions, and less weight will be used for resistance in comparison with programmes that are recommended for beginners without chronic diseases. Encouraging regular exercise of arms, paravertebral muscles and abdominal cavities help in daily tasks and posture during work and leisure [12].

3.2.2 Flexibility exercises

When exercises are performed three times per week, they complement the localized exercise programme. These exercises allow the increase on mobility in a range of joints, not only those affected by connective tissue diseases. Because of the adverse clinical conditions, the movements should provide increased joint range, however, without forcing, in a steady manner. Instead of repetitions, the patient will hold the position for 15 seconds. There is no need to repeat each exercise more than five times for each position because this yields no significant gain.

The improved flexibility benefits the load distribution on the joint cartilage, while the increased range of motion encourages nutrition of the cartilage, an effect that occurs mainly in the synovial joints because of improved circulation and distribution of the synovial fluid. This increased mobility brings patients' independence in their daily lives and can inspire other activities such as dance, yoga and tai chi, for example [11, 12].

4. Coordination, balance and proprioception exercises

Although it is fundamental to health, coordination is not addressed in specific programmes, except in situations in which the disease worsens and rehabilitation requires it. The patient will have more strength and flexibility to coordinate movements, which previously was difficult and was abandoned or even avoided. Skill and specific coordination can be trained simultaneously with more complex exercises to train strength and flexibility, for example. Exercises that involve balance, coordination and proprioception prevent falls, which can be disastrous in this group of patients [13].

5. Speed

In general, in the treatment of degenerative diseases with exercises, the speed that movements and activities are executed will emerge as a direct consequence of advances in the physical capacity for exercise.

6. Method preferred by the author, according to the literature

The sequence of exercises presented below was designed and used to treat degenerative arthritis of the knee after trauma with impairment of the articular cartilage, which required surgical treatment. After the postoperative period was complete and physical therapy was administered for rehabilitation (while pain and functional disability were still present), patients have begun to be part of the study group for this research [14, 15].

To all patients, pain decreased with the use of hyaluronic acid in an intra-articular infusion. Assessment by a doctor of sports medicine has determined the appropriate thresholds for intensity, duration, frequency and type of exercise. In the following example, the patient was able to perform all of the suggested activities in the weekly volume presented.

The aerobic training involved walks four times per week in 30-minute sessions at an intensity determined by stress tests by the ability to chat or hum or by the heart rate determined by the attending physician through mathematical formulas, always corresponding to 50% of $VO2_{max}$. The walks were to always take place on flat terrain with only a few gentle curves. The direction of walking was to be reversed (clockwise to counterclockwise and vice versa) every 10 minutes.

6.1 Suggested exercises

Once the patient was warmed up (through aerobic activity or independently), the exercises described below were performed three times per week, with at least 1 day between sessions for better recovery and utilization.

6.1.1 Lying on your back (supine position)

With one leg bent and the other extended, place a strap on the foot and lift the leg, keeping the knee extended and the ankle at 90°. Hold the position still for 15 seconds (without forcing), and return to the resting position for 5 seconds. Next, repeat the same motion with the other leg. Perform five repetitions for each leg, at intervals of 15 seconds of exercise and 5 seconds of recovery (**Figure 1**).

6.1.2 Lying on your belly (prone position)

Bend one of your knees, and keep the other extended. Holding the ankle and leg with the knee bent, count 15 seconds and then relax, returning to the rest position (**Figure 2**). In some cases, the joint may not permit full flexion; use a strap to maintain a lesser degree of knee flexion while the position is maintained (**Figure 3**). Perform five repetitions for each leg, at intervals of 15 seconds of exercise and 5 seconds of recovery.

6.1.3 Lying on your back (supine position)

Bend one leg at the knee, and support the foot. The other leg should be extended with a soft support under the other knee (a rolled towel or foam pad). Force this extended knee down, pressing against the ground, holding for 20 seconds in isometric contraction. Then, relax for 5 seconds. Repeat 10 times for each leg in two sets totalling 20 repetitions (**Figure 4**).

6.1.4 Lying on your back (supine position)

Bend one leg at the knee, and extend the other leg. The same support used in the previous exercise will be placed under the heel of the extended leg, maintaining

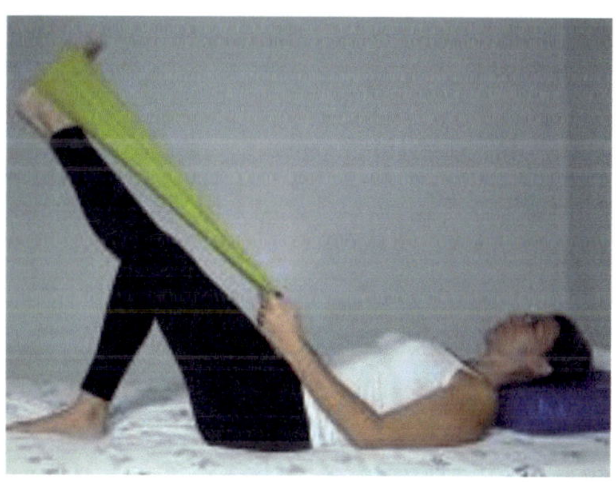

Figure 1.
Stretching back muscles.

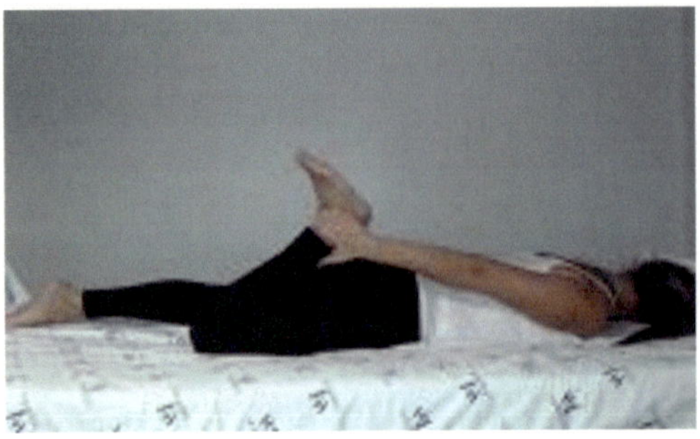

Figure 2.
Stretching previous muscles.

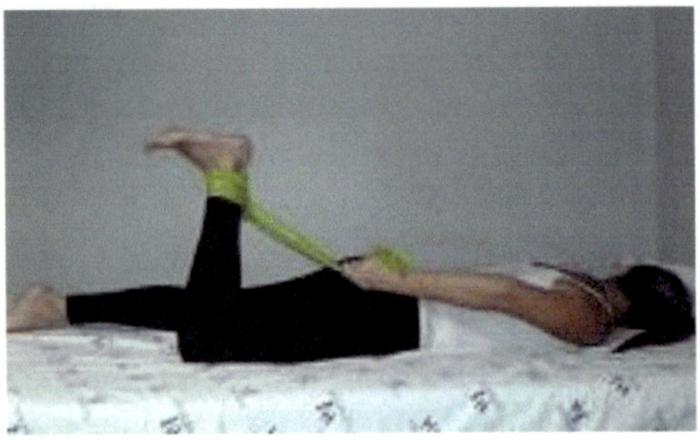

Figure 3.
Strengthening of anterior muscles.

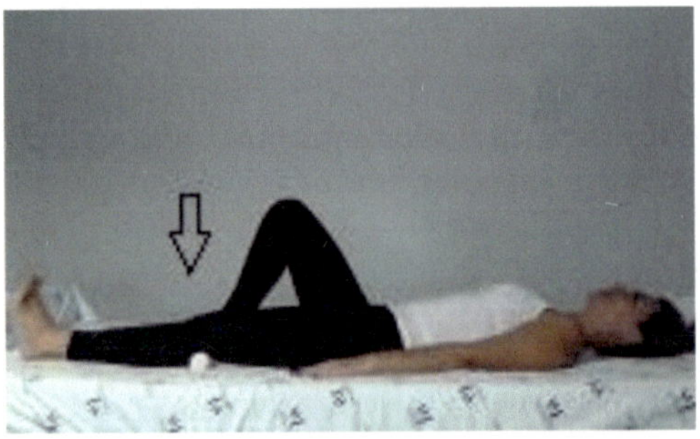

Figure 4.
Isometric contraction for thigh.

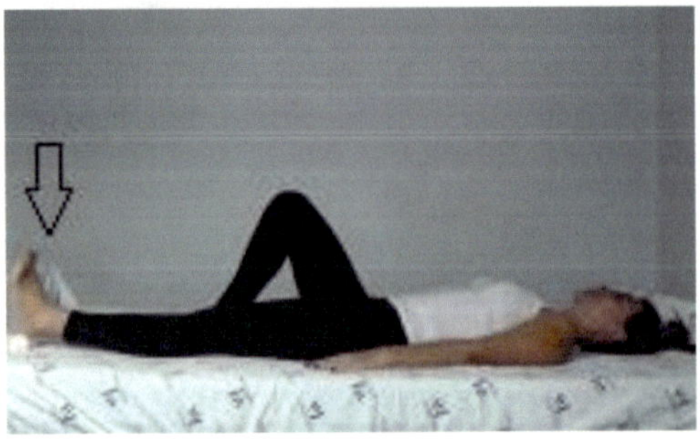

Figure 5.
Isometric contraction for leg.

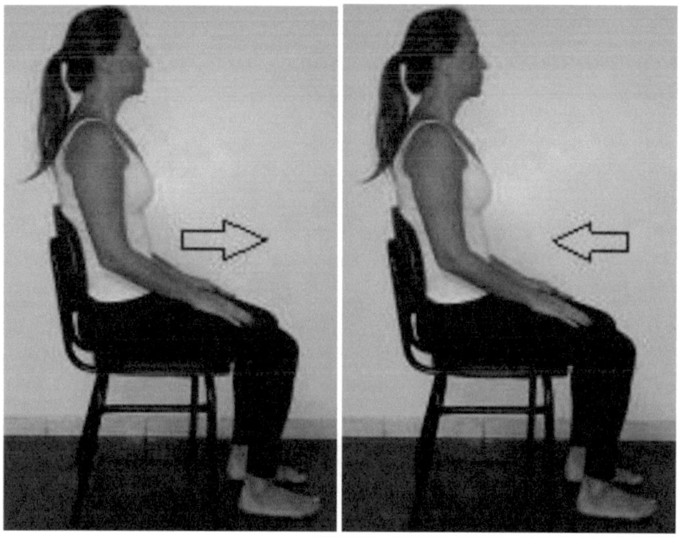

Figure 6.
Abdomen strengthening.

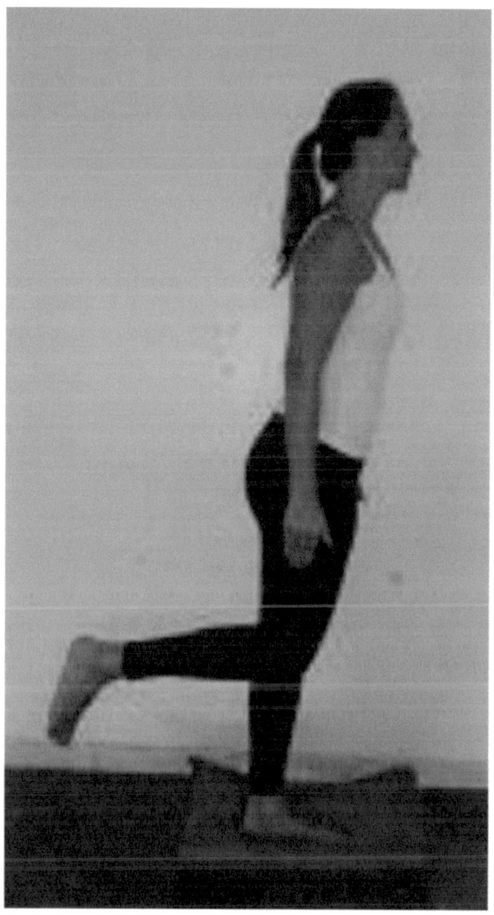

Figure 7.
Exercise for simple body balance.

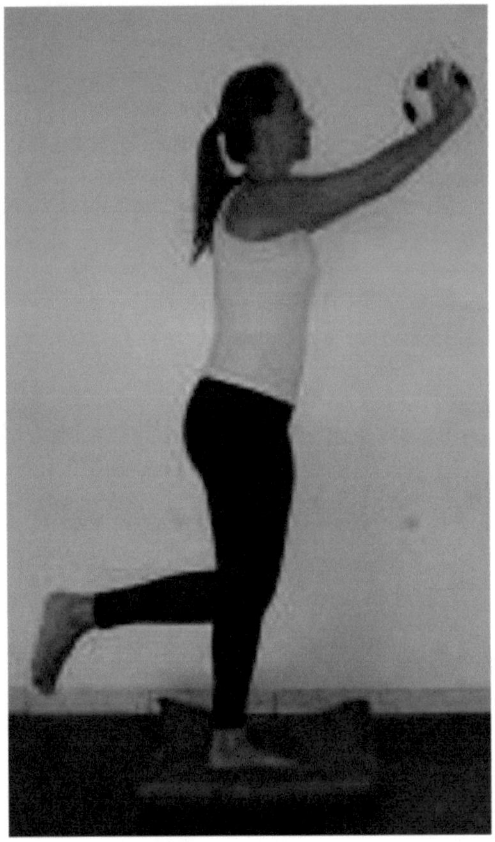

Figure 8.
Exercise for advanced body balance.

pressure against the ground for 20 seconds in isometric contraction. Relax for 5 seconds and repeat the movement with the other leg (**Figure 5**).

6.1.5 Sit in a chair with your back (lumbar region)

Supported and knees flexed at 90° and feet fully supported by the ground or on a support. In this position, flex your muscles as if it was to move the chair forwards (without actually moving the chair forwards), and hold this position for 20 seconds; then relax for 5 seconds. Next, move your muscles as if it was to move the chair backwards (again, without actually moving the chair), and hold this position for 20 seconds, again followed by a rest period of 5 seconds. Perform 10 repetitions for the combined "chair movements" (**Figure 6**).

6.1.6 Standing on a cushion (or foam support)

Try to balance yourself on only one leg; stay close to a wall or some means of support, in case you lose your balance. Flex and extend your hips, knees and ankles to a small extent without losing the position, and keep your eyes fixed on the horizon. This exercise should be performed for a full minute, one leg each minute (**Figure 7**). When you feel safe with regard to balance and executing the movements described above, repeat for another minute, but this time throw a ball against the wall or support, always maintaining your posture and your gaze at the horizon (**Figure 8**).

7. Discussion

We live in an era in which sedentarism has become one of the leading causes of morbidity and mortality. For patients with CDH, such as RA, PM, DM, and SS, phobia due to the pain associated with these diseases may lead to greater immobility, more pain, greater body weight (obesity) leading to more immobility and so on. Entering this vicious circle, patients with CTD will have their activities compromised, such as getting up from a chair, going up and down stairs, shorter walks and difficulty in doing housework. Once the limitations that go beyond the underlying disease are established, patients are dependent on family members or specialized professionals, which makes their lives totally dependent [16].

Regular aerobic exercises and muscle strengthening exercises mainly in the affected joints may interrupt the pain cycle in patients with RA. The review promoted by Hurkmans [9, 17] showed that this association can improve the pain and functional capacity of the locomotor system. It has also been shown that the adaptations occur rapidly and that there is no additional damage to the joints and other tissues affected by the CTD [17]. The review shows that there is sufficient evidence in the literature to state that the medium in which the exercises are performed does not interfere with the beneficial result obtained. Thus, practising the solo or aquatic exercises did not show differences that justify the choice of one of the two for the patients with CTD [17]. Regular exercises of strength and localized muscular resistance and aerobic exercises have been shown to be ancillary to muscular diseases such as PM and DM when practised in moderate intensity, although they do not present sufficient evidence to support clinical observations. It can be affirmed, however, that the practice occurs totally free of physical damages to the practising patients, the fact that counts on evidence that allows reaching that conclusion [18].

Strength training and aerobic resistance training should include proprioception exercises (balance) alone or not. There is evidence in the literature to conclude about its efficiency in patients with CTD, especially in RA and OA knees, contrary to what was demonstrated. Clinical experience points in the direction that the practice of balance exercises should be part of regular training programmes. Takacs et al. have demonstrated that after training for 10 weeks there is an improvement in pain, function and especially the loss of fear of movement when balancing exercises are performed in isolation. However, the lack of further studies still leaves evidence of its benefits not very well-defined [19–21].

The benefits of regular physical activity and the harm of sedentary lifestyle and its consequences are well demonstrated in the review by Pinto et al. on autoimmune diseases. The advice to sit less and move more (sit less and move more) is also applied to CTA patients. The review definitely shows the benefits that regular physical activity brings to people with autoimmune rheumatic diseases. As to the intensity of the work performed, it was noted that it need not necessarily be intense. Mild exercises can also help these patients. Most of the studies cited, however, advocate on even increasing intensities for those who demonstrate adaptation to the stimulus offered [22].

Additional benefits can be realized in patients with CTD. In their experiment, Stavropoulos-Kalinoglou et al. demonstrated that aerobic and localized muscular endurance exercises reduce the risk of cardiovascular diseases in patients with RA besides increasing their physical work capacity. It also showed that when the prescriptions are individualized, works at lower intensities produce a protective effect as well as those of greater intensity in those who had restrictions for such [23].

8. Conclusion

Regular physical activity yields countless benefits to patients with degenerative diseases of the connective tissue, both in terms of prevention and in association with a treatment regimen.

The intensity, duration, frequency and type of exercises should be determined by each clinical condition of the patient, and it should be studied on a case-by-case basis for individualized recommendations.

Author details

Ricardo Munir Nahas[1,2*], Vivianne Horsti Dos Santos[3] and Silvio Lopes Alabarse[4,5]

1 Center of Medicine of the Exercise and Sports of Nove de Julho Hospital, Director and Orthopedic Surgeon, São Paulo, Brazil

2 Assistance Management of Ipiranga Public Hospital, São Paulo, Brazil

3 Data Analyst, University of Kent, United Kingdom

4 Professor at the University of Mogi das, Cruzes

5 Researcher at the Federal University of, São Paulo

*Address all correspondence to: rmnahas@uol.com.br

References

[1] Nagy G, Huszthy PC, Fossum E, Konttinen Y, Nakken B, Szodoray P. Selected aspects in the pathogenesis of autoimmune diseases. Mediators of Inflammation. 2015;**2015**:1-11. DOI: 10.1155/2015/351732

[2] Azukizawa M, Ito H, Hamamoto Y, Fujii T, Morita Y, Okahata A, et al. The effects of well-rounded exercise program on systemic biomarkers related to cartilage metabolism. Cartilage. 2018;**2018**:1-8. DOI: 10.1177/19476035187679

[3] Smith BE, Hendrick P, Smith TO, Bateman M, Moffatt F, Rathleff MS, et al. Should exercises be painful in the management of chronic musculoskeletal pain? A systematic review and meta-analysis. British Journal of Sports Medicine. 2017;**51**(23):1679-1687. DOI: 10.1136/bjsports-2016-097383

[4] Moseng T, Dagfinrud H, Smedslund G, Østerås N. The importance of dose in land-based supervised exercise for people with hip osteoarthritis. A systematic review and meta-analysis. Osteoarthritis and Cartilage. 2017;**25**(10):1563-1576. DOI: 10.1016/j.joca.2017.06.004

[5] Egan B, Zierath JR. Exercise metabolism and the molecular regulation of skeletal muscle adaptation. Cell Metabolism. 2013;**17**:162-184. DOI: 10.1016/j.cmet.2012.12.012

[6] Barrès R, Yan J, Egan B, Treebak JT, Rasmussen M, Fritz T, et al. Acute exercise remodels promoter methylation in human skeletal muscle. Cell Metabolism. 2012;**15**(3):405-411. DOI: 10.1016/j.cmet.2012.01.001

[7] Segan JD, Briggs AM, Chou L, Connelly KL, Seneviwickrama M, Sullivan K, et al. Patient-perceived health service needs in inflammatory arthritis: A systematic scoping review seminars in arthritis and rheumatism 2017. Seminars in Arthritis and Rheumatism. 2018;**47**(6):765-777. DOI: 10.1016/j.semarthrit.2017.10.019

[8] Sveaas SH, Smedslund G, Hagen KB, Dagfinrud H. Effect of cardiorespiratory and strength exercises on disease activity in patients with inflammatory rheumatic diseases: A systematic review and meta-analysis. British Journal of Sports Medicine;**51**:1065-1072. DOI: 10.1136/bjsports-2016-097149 2017

[9] Metsios GS, Stavropoulos-Kalinoglou A, Kitas GD. The role of exercise in the management of rheumatoid arthritis. Expert Review of Clinical Immunology. 2015;**11**(10):1121-1130. DOI: 10.1586/1744666X.2015.1067606.2015

[10] Giannotti E, Koutsikos K, Pigatto M, Rampudda ME, Doria A, Masiero S. Medium-/long-term effects of a specific exercise protocol combined with patient education on spine mobility, chronic fatigue, pain, aerobic fitness and level of disability in fibromyalgia. BioMed Research International. 2014;**2014**:474029. DOI: 10.1155/2014/474029

[11] Bernard P, Hains-Monfette G, Atoui S, Kingsbury C. Differences in daily objective physical activity and sedentary time between women with self-reported fibromyalgia and controls: Results from the Canadian health measures survey. Clinical Rheumatology. 2018:2285-2290. DOI: 10.1007/s10067-018-4139-6

[12] Sharif K, Watad A, Bragazzi NL, Lichtbroun M, Amital H, Shoenfeld Y. Physical activity and autoimmune diseases: Get moving and manage the disease. Autoimmunity Reviews. 2017;**17**(1):53-72. DOI: 10.1016/j.autrev.2017.11.010

[13] Schiphof D, van den Driest JJ, Runhaar J. Osteoarthritis year in

review 2017: Rehabilitation and outcomes. Osteoarthritis and Cartilage. 2018;**26**(3):326-340. DOI: 10.1016/j.joca.2018.01.006

[14] Wang C, Schmid CH, Fielding RA, Harvey WF, Reid KF, Price LL, et al. Effect of tai chi versus aerobic exercise for fibromyalgia: Comparative effectiveness randomized controlled trial. BMJ. 2018;**360**:k851. DOI: 10.1136/bmj.k851

[15] Nilsen TS, Scott JM, Michalski M, Capaci C, Thomas S, Herndon JE, et al. Jones LW novel methods for reporting of exercise dose and adherence: An exploratory analysis. Medicine and Science in Sports and Exercise. 2018;**50**(6):1134-1141. DOI: 10.1249/MSS.0000000000001545

[16] Vincent HK, Heywood K, Connelly J, Hurley RW. Weight loss and obesity in the treatment and prevention of osteoarthritis. American Academy of Physical Medicine and Rehabilitation. 2012:S59-S67. DOI: 10.1016/j.pmrj.2012.01.005

[17] Hurkmans E, van der Giesen FJ, Vliet Vlieland TPM, Schoones J, Van den Ende ECHM. Dynamic exercise programs (aerobic capacity and/or muscle strength training) in patients with rheumatoid arthritis. The Cochrane Collaboration. 2009

[18] Voet NBM, van der Kooi EL, Riphagen II, Lindeman E, van Engelen BGM, Geurts ACH. Strength training or comprehensive aerobic exercise training for muscle disease. The Cochrane Collaboration. 2013:1-4

[19] Nahas RM, Porto LCK, Ikemoto RY, Tenório FA, Zílio G, Costa RA, et al. Viscosupplementation in the treatment of post-traumatic arthritis of the knee for 12 months. Revista Brasileira de Medicina do Esporte. 2016;**22**(6). DOI: 10.1590/1517-869220162206167840

[20] Silva KNG, Mizusaki Imoto A, Almeida GJM, Atallah ÁN, Peccin MS, Fernandes Moça Trevisani V. Balance training (proprioceptive training) for rheumatoid arthritis. The Cochrane Collaboration. 2010:1-14

[21] Takacs J, Krowchuk NM, Garland SJ, Carpenter MG, Hunt MA. Dynamic balance training improves physical function in individuals with knee osteoarthritis: A pilot randomized controlled trial. American Congress of Rehabilitation Medicine. 2017:1586-1593. DOI: 10.1016/j.apmr.2017.01.029

[22] Pinto AJ, de Sá Pinto AL, Lima FR, Pereira RMR, Silva CA, Bonfá E, et al. Physical inactivity and sedentary behaviour: Overlooked risk factors in autoimmune rheumatic diseases. Autoimmunity Reviews. 2017;**16**(7): 667-674. DOI: 10.1016/i.autrev.2017.05.001

[23] Stavropoulos-Kalinoglou A, Metsios GS, Veldhuijzen van Zanten JJ, Nightingale P, Kitas GD, Koutedakis Y. Individualised aerobic and resistance exercise training improves cardiorespiratory fitness and reduces cardiovascular risk in patients with rheumatoid arthritis. Annals of the Rheumatic Diseases. 2013;**72**(11):1819-1825. DOI: 10.1136/annrheumdis-2012-202075